Detox For Dummies®

Why Detox?

- **Poor diet,** high in fat and refined starches a... sugars, and low in fibre, vitamins, minerals, and *trace elements* (minerals required in tiny quantities).

- **Exposure to cigarette smoke**, which most people inhale whether they are smokers or not.

- **Heavy drinking** – this depends upon the individual, but basically it means drinking more than the Government-recommended amount (14 units per week for women, 21 units per week for men, with 1 unit being a 100 mls standard-strength wine, half a pint of beer, a schooner of sherry, or a single measure of spirits). Heavy drinking is also taking more than 2–3 units per day, and drinking every day without an alcohol break.

- **Caffeine** from highly caffeinated coffee and fizzy drinks.

- **Stress** (which everyone is subject to – see Chapter 8) gives rise to toxic *free radicals* – hyperactive oxygen molecules that attack the immune system, hastening the development of degenerative disorders.

- **Environmental pollutants** such as chlorine in drinking water, traffic emissions, and so on.

How to Avoid the Need for Salt

You can grow accustomed to 'saltlessness' by doctoring vegetables, eggs, meat, and other savouries with fresh or dried herbs, condiments, and spices. Here are some suggestions:

- Add a little English mustard to boiled or mashed potatoes just before serving.

- Use garlic for potatoes, spinach, peas, beans, and other pulses.

- Sprinkle caraway seeds on cabbage and spring greens.

- Try low sodium tomato ketchup or salsa with cauliflower.

- Spice up root vegetables with nutmeg or cinnamon.

- Use low-sodium soy sauce in practically everything.

For Dummies: Bestselling Book Series for Beginners

Glycaemic Index of Select Foods

Food	G.I. Rating	Food	G.I. Rating
Apples	38	Lentils	29
Apricots	57	Skimmed milk	32
French baguette	95	Whole milk	27
Organic baked beans	42	Oats	58
Bananas	52	Oranges	42
Barley	25	Parsnips	97
Butter beans	36	White pasta	40
Haricot beans	38	Wholemeal pasta	37
Kidney beans	29	Peaches	42
Soy beans	15	Peanuts	14
White bread	70	Peas	51
Wholegrain rye bread	42	Popcorn (low fat)	53
Wholegrain wheat bread	77	Baked potatoes	85
Carrots	47	Sweet potatoes	54
Chick peas	42	Raisins	64
Cornflakes	81	Brown rice	55
Grapefruit	25	White rice	74
Grapes	46	Sweetcorn	55
Honey	55	Weetabix	68

Copyright © 2007 John Wiley & Sons, Ltd.
All rights reserved. Item 1908-5.
For more information about John Wiley & Sons,
call (+44) 1243 779777.

For Dummies: Bestselling Book Series for Beginners

Detox FOR DUMMIES®

by Caroline Shreeve

John Wiley & Sons, Ltd

Detox For Dummies®

Published by
John Wiley & Sons, Ltd
The Atrium
Southern Gate
Chichester
West Sussex
PO19 8SQ
England

E-mail (for orders and customer service enquires): cs-books@wiley.co.uk

Visit our Home Page on www.wileyeurope.com

Copyright © 2007 John Wiley & Sons, Ltd, Chichester, West Sussex, England

Published by John Wiley & Sons, Ltd, Chichester, West Sussex

Wiley also publishes its books in a variety of electronic formats. Some content that appears in print may not be available in electronic books.

British Library Cataloguing in Publication Data: A catalogue record for this book is available from the British Library.

ISBN-13: 978-0-470-01908-5

Printed and bound in Great Britain by TJ International, Padstow, Cornwall

10 9 8 7 6 5 4 3 2

WILEY

About the Author

Caroline Shreeve is a GP with a particular interest in nutrition and complementary medicine. She has written magazine articles and books about both, as well as about orthodox medicine, and frequently advises her patients about dietary measures to help relieve and cure a variety of ailments.

She has discovered the usefulness of detox both for herself and others in her care, and is an enthusiastic supporter of nutritional supplements, in appropriate situations and in safe quantities. She has researched the effects of toxins on the immune defence system since the 1980s, together with the benefits of antioxidants to counteract the effects of free radical damage.

Caroline has lived and worked in South Africa, the (then) Transkei and Australia, and lectured on nutritional and related topics in Australia, New Zealand, and many European countries. She now lives and works in rural West Wales, where she lives with her two pugs and several rescue cats.

Publisher's Acknowledgements

We're proud of this book; please send us your comments through our Dummies online registration form located at www.dummies.com/register/.

Some of the people who helped bring this book to market include the following:

Acquisitions, Editorial, and Media Development

Executive Project Editor: Martin Tribe

Content Editor: Steve Edwards

Commissioning Editor: Alison Yates

Development Editor: Kathleen Dobie

Copy Editor: Martin Key

Proofreader: Kim Vernon

Technical Editor: Maria Griffiths Dip ION, BANT www.familynutritioninpractice.com

Recipe Tester: Emily Nolan

Executive Editor: Jason Dunne

Cover Photo: Don Farrall/Getty Images

Cartoons: Ed McLachlan

Composition

Project Coordinator: Jennifer Theriot

Layout and Graphics: Claudia Bell, Denny Hager, Stephanie D. Jumper, Heather Ryan, Alicia South

Proofreaders: Amanda Briggs, David Faust, Charles Spencer, Brian H. Walls

Indexer: Techbooks

Publishing and Editorial for Consumer Dummies

    Diane Graves Steele, Vice President and Publisher, Consumer Dummies

    Joyce Pepple, Acquisitions Director, Consumer Dummies

    Kristin A. Cocks, Product Development Director, Consumer Dummies

    Michael Spring, Vice President and Publisher, Travel

    Kelly Regan, Editorial Director, Travel

Publishing for Technology Dummies

    Andy Cummings, Vice President and Publisher, Dummies Technology/General User

Composition Services

    Gerry Fahey, Vice President of Production Services

    Debbie Stailey, Director of Composition Services

Contents at a Glance

Table of Contents

Introduction

● ●

*W*elcome to *Detox For Dummies!* One of my aims in writing this book has been to clarify the main issues of the detox process, and, hopefully, to explain how it works in such as a way that you'll be planning your own detox by the time you finish reading it.

You probably know a little about detox already, having read of its use by celebrities, and its inclusion in spa health regimens, which generally come at a high price. But there is so much more to detox than an ability to remove pounds of 'baby fat' from a woman shortly after giving birth, and ridding sufferers of unsightly cellulite. In fact, these aspects are mentioned only in passing in this book, because I believe that they obscure the fundamental health benefits that are available to all those seeking improved health and vitality.

About This Book

The thrust of this book is detox's strengthening action on your immune defence system. In ridding your body of stored poisons, you are freeing your immune cells to perform their intended task. This, primarily, is to counteract the destructive effect of free radicals – hyperactive oxygen fragments that develop in the tissues in response to toxin exposure.

When allowed to accumulate, free radicals cause many undesirable effects – premature ageing (including lines and wrinkles), for example, and degenerative disorders such as cancer, arthritis, and immune complaints. Hay fever, asthma, allergies, and eczema are all common examples.

I hope you enjoy this book as much as I have enjoyed writing it. You can be sure of reading about many detox benefits that the popular press generally forgets to mention. You'll also discover that, whoever and wherever you are, you can organise your own personal detox to suit *you* as an individual, at very little cost and effort.

Foolish Assumptions

This book makes certain educated guesses about you. Rightly or wrongly, this book assumes that:

- ✔ You have never detoxed before and want to know more about the detox process.
- ✔ You are basically healthy, and are neither pregnant nor suffering from an eating disorder.
- ✔ You are open-minded to the benefits detox has to offer.

How This Book Is Organised

The following section sets out the plan I have used to organise this book. I believe that understanding the basic principles of detoxing is important if you are to set out on a detox plan of your own design aimed at achieving certain goals. However, I do try to avoid too much technical detail, providing, instead, clear, everyday examples which are easy to relate to.

Part 1: Detox Basics

In this part I explain the fundamental principles of detox. I tell you about the three main stages – cleansing, balancing, and fortifying – and how they overlap and complement one another's actions. I'll show you how the principles of detox achieve their health-giving goals, and how you can encourage your personal detox programme to work for best for you.

Part 11: Detoxing Your Diet

Some foods are advisable to avoid during detox. I show you those to avoid when detoxing – and, hopefully, continue to avoid in the future (except in small quantities). Equally importantly, I go into detail about the foods to choose (and why) when detoxing, and for the sake of good health generally.

Part 111: Detoxing Your Lifestyle

Detoxing is a lifestyle choice. I look at many aspects of lifestyles and of life generally. I point out common, often unsuspected, sources of toxins and suggest how you can avoid them.

Part IV: Planning Your Detox

Here I'll show you how to plan your own detox. Customising your detox programme is important to success, and examples are given of detox programmes of varying length, from a couple of days to two weeks in length.

Part V: Delicious Detox Recipes

This part shows that detox foods need not be boring and provides six chapters of delectable recipes covering every aspect of eating during your detox. I offer many choices and explain how to select the meals best suited to your own personal lifestyle.

Part VI: The Part of Tens

This part divides some of the key information on managing your detox into lists, each containing ten 'information bites'. I include ten therapies that can help enhance detox, ten myths about detox, and ten tips to help you stay motivated.

Icons Used in This Book

The icons tell you what you must know, what you should know, and what you may find interesting but can live without.

When you see this icon, it means the information is essential, and you should pay attention to it.

This icon marks important information that can save you time and energy.

The Warning icon cautions you against potential problems.

You gain from this information, but if you do decide to ignore it you aren't putting your detox at risk.

Where to Go from Here

If you're close to committing to a detox, but can't quite give your-self the oomph you need, then check out toxins and their sources in Chapter 2, and the basics of detoxing in Chapter 4. If you're still not quite there, take a look at Chapter 20 (Ten Myths About Detox), and read, in Chapter 5, about the delectable foods you'll be eating. Firm up your resolution with the recipes in Chapters 13 through 18.

Part I
Detox Basics

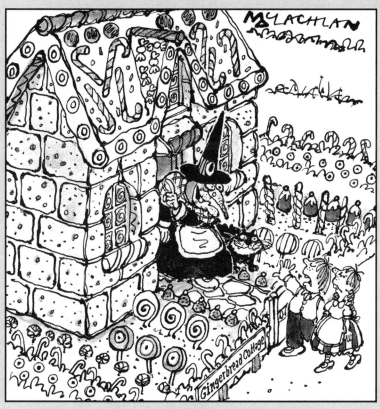

"No thanks — we're detoxing."

In this part . . .

*H*ere I cover what detox is all about. In Chapter 1 I explain detox principles and how the process benefits health and vitality.

In Chapter 2 I describe many common toxins, some of which you may be familiar with, while others may be lurking in your food, home, or other environment without your even having heard of them.

In Chapter 3 I tell you about your detox organs: Liver, kidneys, bowel, lungs, and skin, including how they work hard for you 24/7 to rid your system of toxic substances. Equally importantly, I explain how you can support them and keep them labouring happily on your behalf.

Chapter 1

Figuring Out What Detox Is All About

This chapter gives you an overview of detox: what it is and who can benefit from it. Importantly, it also covers who should *not* detox.

Everyone is different, and every detox plan is different in the sense that your personal choices have to be right for *you*. Above all, I encourage you to plan the detox that best suits you as an individual.

Examining Detox Basics

What exactly is detox? *Detox* is the process of ridding the body of *toxins* – harmful substances that accumulate in the organs and tissues.

Encountering toxins

Toxins are all around you, cropping up occasionally where you least expect them.

This book aims to help you understand that most damaging substances don't come with big DANGER signs attached (more on this in Chapter 2).

Some toxins, such as petrol fumes and insecticides, obviously have toxic properties, but not all the injurious substances targeted by a detox plan are toxic in the accepted sense of the word. Take tartrazine, for example. This yellow dye – found in biscuits, cakes, drinks, and other edibles – is not a poison, as such – it will not kill you, or even make you ill. However, many studies carried out since the 1980s link its consumption with attention deficit hyperactivity disorder, which impairs the concentration of children of all ages, and causes poor sleeping habits, unruly – even violent – behaviour, and the feeling of being in a state of perpetual motion.

Junk snacks and convenience foods contain artificial preservatives, colourings, and flavourings with no nutritional value and lots of toxic potential.

Living the vida toxic

A toxic lifestyle consists of one (and maybe all) of the following:

- ✔ A **poor diet,** high in fat and refined starches and sugars and low in fibre, vitamins, minerals, and *trace elements* (minerals required in tiny quantities).

- ✔ Exposure to **cigarette smoke,** which most people inhale whether they are smokers or not.

- ✔ **Heavy drinking** – this depends upon the individual, but basically it means drinking more than the Government-recommended amount (14 units per week for women, 21 units per week for men, with 1 unit being a 100 mls standard strength wine, half a pint of beer, a schooner of sherry, or a single measure of spirits). Heavy drinking is also taking more than 2–3 units per day, and drinking every day without an alcohol break.

- ✔ **Caffeine** from highly caffeinated coffee and fizzy drinks.

- ✔ **Stress** (which everyone is subject to – see Chapter 8) gives rise to toxic *free radicals* – hyperactive oxygen molecules that attack the immune system, hastening the development of degenerative disorders.

- ✔ **Environmental pollutants** such as chlorine in drinking water, traffic emissions, and so on.

All the above toxic exposures impair the immune defence system, and their combined effects have proven links to heart and arterial disease, cancer, diabetes, premature ageing, and other degenerative disorders.

Chronic toxin overload is the state you get into if you never bother to counteract these effects with detox.

Everyone is susceptible to toxin overload, which can harm you directly – for example, a high alcohol intake leading to liver cirrhosis – and indirectly by weakening the immune defence system (see Chapter 3).

Turning to the bright side

It may seem that everything you enjoy, or use to relieve stress, is full of toxins. The good news is that many substances with toxic potential when taken in large quantities, such as chocolate and alcohol, can be perfectly safe or even health-promoting when taken in moderation.

The even better news is that detoxing can cleanse, balance, and fortify your system (see the next section), eliminate many stored 'nasties' and decrease your chances of suffering at their hands.

Going through the Process

Although I describe the cleansing, balancing and restorative stages of detox (see Chapter 4) in sequence, each is more or less ongoing and merges seamlessly with the next. Cleansing does not screech to a halt, for example, when you start balancing, nor does balancing slam its brakes on when you start fortifying. The idea is to work with nature, not frighten it to death!

Cleansing

The cleansing stage encourages your excretory organs – your liver, kidneys, gut, lungs, and skin – to get rid of toxins, big time. Fibre-rich foods, for example, help your bowels to work, while the extra fluid washes out water-soluble toxins in your urine.

You may decide to kick off with a 'liquids only' day, taking only water and freshly-squeezed juices. (Chapter 4 talks about whether to start your detox plan in this way or go straight on with the recommended foods – such as organic fruit, vegetables, grains, pulses – that nourish and support the cleansing process.)

Going with organic foods

Chapter 5 has more about the benefits of choosing organic produce, and I'll just say at this point that organically grown veg and fruit contain on average twice the vitamins, minerals, trace elements, essential fatty acids, and plant nutrients of non-organic produce – and in their natural ratios.

Fresh or frozen vegetables and fruit have their full complement of fibre, a great, natural-bulking agent which helps your bowels to work fully and regularly. Soluble and insoluble fibre also absorbs many of the toxins on their way out of your intestinal system, buffering the bowel lining against any irritation these toxins may cause.

Your liver, kidneys, skin, gut, and lungs need all the nutritional support you can give them when they are working hard to eject long-stored toxins.

Keying in on chelating foods

A natural bodily process called *chelation (key'lation)* neutralises and takes out toxic metals such as lead and mercury.

A number of nutrients encourage chelation, of which vitamin C is probably the most important. Vitamin C cannot be stored by the body because this vitamin is water-soluble and, as readily as your gut absorbs it from fresh fruit and vegetables, it is excreted in the urine.

This is one reason why a constant supply of vitamin C–rich fruit and veg and certain other foods play such an important role in detox plans.

Chapter 5 talks about your food choices to aid detox cleansing, and you can find recipes utilising them in Chapters 13 to 18. Chapter 6 tells you about the foods to avoid when detoxing, and the reasons why.

Balancing

The object of the balancing stage of detox is to re-balance your body nutritionally after establishing the cleansing stage. You eat the same foods, but with a wider choice and generally more protein.

Central to the re-balancing process is the addition of herbal and nutritional supplements (apart from antioxidant minerals and vitamins, and acidophilus sources). Favourite balancing herbs (detailed in Chapter 11) include the adaptogens such as ginseng which help your body to 'adapt to' and benefit fully from the detox process. They also give you the strength to cope with stress and illnesses in the future.

Re-balancing nutritional supplements include omega-6 essential fatty acids found in evening primrose oil, and the omega-3 group supplied by fish oils.

Fortifying

Once cleansing and balancing are underway, and you're countering stress with simple exercise and relaxation, detox fortifying helps to strengthen you against further toxins.

The choice of foods and recipes are widened, and you are eased gradually back into a healthy eating plan which improves your energy and stamina forthwith.

Supplements can help you with detox fortifying, and I discuss them in Chapter 11.

Offering Reasons to Detox

People detox for a variety of reasons, especially those in the following sections.

Detoxing for weight loss

You are likely to lose weight when detoxing, partly because healthy, natural foods contain far less saturated fat and sugar and provide fewer calories. Another reason may be more regular bowel movements. If you're not usually 'regular', but have to take laxatives to open your bowels once or twice a week (for instance), your colon may be clogged with a hefty waste overload. Until you shift this and spring-clean your gut, satisfactory weight loss won't happen. You can help the process along, and benefit from longer-lasting weight loss, with the use of certain supplements (such as psyllium husks – an excellent inner gut 'broom'), which help gut balancing and activity by providing helpful bacteria, which every large bowel needs! These supplements are discussed in Chapter 11.

If you do not suffer from constipation but can't shed weight, ask your doctor to check your general health and look beyond detox (to cutting your calorie intake or becoming more active, for instance) for a realistic loss.

Detoxing for health

You may be considering a detox to boost your general health, though you feel in pretty good shape and have no specific symptoms to relieve.

Detoxing boosts your immune defence system, strengthening it to deal with the free radicals that are generated in the tissues through stress and other toxins. Catching fewer colds and similar infections (or getting over them more quickly), the more rapid healing of minor injuries (such as scratches, cuts and bruises), more restful sleep, a fresher complexion, and improved vitality, are just a few additional benefits.

On the other hand, you may turn to detox to relieve minor conditions. Degenerative problems such as premature ageing (masses of wrinkles and lines), arthritis or poor circulation, small skin cancers, and 'borderline' diabetes all spring to mind.

Alternatively, you may wish to strengthen your immune system because you're prone to allergic disorders – eczema, asthma, and hayfever, for instance.

 Seek medical advice from your doctor if you are receiving ongoing treatment. Otherwise, your symptoms are likely to improve, and you'll feel encouraged to, and I recommend that you do, detox several times a year.

Detoxing for energy

Has your get-up-and-go got up and gone? Prolonged stress, long working hours, anxiety over finances, relationships or family members, above all toxin overload, can sap your energy, leaving you exhausted and irritable. You're left with zilch interest in sex – or any other pleasures for that matter.

Though you may feel tempted to smoke or drink too much to ease your unpleasant state, listen to your body, and try detoxing instead.

The cleansing stage puts paid to accumulated toxins and gathered waste matter, the balancing process re-harmonises your over-stressed system (and immune defences), and you can then fortify yourself physically and mentally with highly nutritional foods.

 Essential to your plan is gentle exercise and regular relaxation to help you get rid of negative emotions and fight depression. Besides boosting your mood, they also provide physical and mental repose.

Mood, anxiety levels, and sleep quality tend to improve fairly quickly. You need to continue your healthy diet (and stress-beating measures) to benefit in the long-term.

Planning Your Personal Detox

You have decided to detox – it's just a question of when and where. However enthusiastic you may feel, though, being in the right mood, in the right place, and at the right time is just as essential to your ultimate success as eating the recommended foods and drinking lots of water.

Getting in the mood

Your mood and your stress level are both important factors to consider before starting a detox. You need to feel in a positive, fairly upbeat mood to detox. The first day or so can be challenging, especially if you're a heavy-coffee drinking, party-going smoker who loves a tipple!

See your GP if you think you may be suffering from depression, and check out Chapter 8 to identify stress symptoms.

Finding the right time

New Year is a classic time to detox, following seasonal excesses – there's also the lure of your healthier self sashaying into spring. And springtime lends itself to detoxing, being a time of renewal and growth.

Your body, mind and emotions tell you when to detox, if you listen to them. A holiday is an ideal opportunity, as is a fairly slack week ahead when you've a long weekend with minimum stress and plenty of time to yourself.

You can start by reading Chapter 21 in which I supply ten top tips to keep you motivated.

Staking out the right place

In theory, you can detox anywhere, but your home is probably the best place, where you're in charge of the food and can throw out tempting snacks that definitely aren't on the menu! (See Chapter 6 on which foods to avoid, and why.)

You may feel a hotel or spa is preferable, if there are therapies on hand to keep you on track. But hotels have dishes that just *might* tempt you, and spas, while ostensibly places of tranquillity, may produce unforeseen aggravation beyond your control.

Being prepared

It's advisable to prepare yourself for detoxing, because this important event should ideally set the scene for a healthier future lifestyle. And if you habitually take in a lot of caffeine, sugar or refined, processed foods, you need to cut down on these before your detox starts.

The chapters in Part IV are all about personalising your detox, and making the best choices for *you:*

✔ Chapter 10 helps you every step of the way as you draw up your detox plan, both preparing to detox and actually doing it.

✔ Chapter 11 tells you all about dietary and herbal supplements you can select to optimise your detoxing experience.

✔ Chapter 12 points you in the direction of maintaining detox for life.

Looking at Who Shouldn't Detox

Take time out to listen to your body – it should be spelling out its needs regarding detox, loud and clear. Take a look at Chapter 2, if you are in any doubt about your need to detox.

There are circumstances, however, in which detoxing is a definite no-no, and others in which I would urge you to check with your doctor before planning a detox routine.

Don't detox if

✔ You are pregnant or breast-feeding

✔ You suffer from a serious illness

✔ You will shortly be having an operation

✔ You are grossly over- or underweight and/or suffer from an eating disorder. (This means clinically obese, with a Body Mass Index above 30. To check yours go to nhlbisupport. com/bmi/.)

Always check with your doctor if

✔ You are in any doubt about your fitness to detox (your doctor may not be sure what detoxing is, so take a copy of this book – or a photocopy of your chosen plan – with you!)

✔ You are being treated for any condition with prescription medicines.

Chapter 2

Toxins, Toxins Everywhere

*Y*ou hear a lot about toxins in food these days. Perhaps, at times, too much? Unhealthy substances enter the natural food chain at certain points, being added to processed foods as preservatives, dyes, and flavourings.

Food dubbed a 'superfood' one minute is often condemned the next because it's said to be loaded with noxious substances. How confusing is that? Take salmon, for example. Chock-full of omega-3 essential fatty acids, nutritionists urge you to eat it for the sake of your heart and brains. Then, lo and behold, mercury and other toxins are discovered in commercially farmed salmon (the type most commonly found in supermarkets and the one that most of us can afford) and we're also warned against the dye used to enhance its natural pink colour. Polyunsaturated margarine replaced butter for many of us, once we'd accepted the health risks of saturated fats. Now, we're warned against the trans-fats in plant-derived spreads caused by the high-temperature manufacturing processes (refer to Chapter 1).

'Wolf!' cried too frequently can fall on deaf ears. It's simpler and less stressful to stick with what you know. However, toxins in food and the environment *do* pose genuine health risks and you can counteract much potential damage by learning a bit about them.

Defining Toxins

Toxins are like weeds, the narcissistic thugs of the plant world bent on taking over. Poisonous fungi, ragwort, and columbine threaten the lives of humans, farm animals, and plants respectively so they get rooted up and destroyed. Dandelions, nettles, and couch grass are also doomed – they're valuable herbal remedies, but they ruin herbaceous borders and lawns.

Likewise, certain toxins are out-and-out bad news – petrol and diesel fumes, for instance, tobacco smoke, lead, and aluminium in the water supply, and many food additives, which I get into later in this chapter. Other toxins, such as alcohol, have their benign side. Few regular drinkers would label their favourite poison . . . well, poisonous (except during a hangover). Indeed, rum has provided vital warmth and cheer to centuries of sailors.

As you read in Chapter 1, toxins for the purpose of a detox, are substances that accumulate in the body and cause it harm. Toxins include lead from old paint and ancient plumbing, aluminium from cooking utensils, and petrol fumes. Other less obvious ones are the hydrogenated fats used in processed foods and junk snacks.

Recent scientific evidence has even shown that real ale and red wine offer some protection against heart attacks and strokes. Conversely, alcoholism claims millions of lives yearly, and binge drinking fuels up to 80 per cent of crime and yobbish behaviour.

Toxin definition also comes down to perception, and also to common sense. The dandelions, couch grass and nettles I mention above can be seen as brutish weeds or basic remedy sources. Tap water in the UK is perfectly safe to drink, except on the rare occasions when it becomes contaminated by a toxin. Domestic central-heating oil, for instance, can trickle from a leaking tank into a nearby stream, toxifying the drinking water of farm animals and plant food crops.

Getting to know the potential harm of certain foods and drinks and the effects of lifestyle choices and habits enables you to make informed choices about what you eat, how you live, and how often you should detox.

Feeling the effects of toxins

Poisonous or waste substances accumulate within your body, over-taxing the organs that work to rid your body of wastes, including your liver, kidneys, bowel, lungs, and skin. This build-up of waste leads to materials being excreted from your body less efficiently than usual. Surplus free radicals are generated, impairing the immune system.

With your immune system below par, you run an increased risk of suffering from major and minor infections, allergies, and degenerative disorders such as arthritis, diabetes, cancer, arterial disease and dementia. Food intolerances are often the cause of an impaired immune system.

When your body is dealing with an overload of toxins, you may experience any of the following:

- Bad taste in the mouth, bad breath
- Spotty, greasy skin and pasty complexion
- Bloating and weight gain
- Fatigue, poor sleep, lethargy
- Aching muscles and joints
- Strongly smelling urine not caused by infection
- Sluggish bowel movements.

Effective bowel motions are essential to health, but it is equally important to avoid becoming fixated on the subject. Healthy bowels work like clockwork, according to laxative manufacturers, and also to the minority of people who can (and doubtless do) set the watches by the post-breakfast evacuation.

The truth is that bowels, like their owners, are individuals, which means that what is 'right' for you and, say, a couple of other people with whom you've compared notes, is probably not right at all for your next-door neighbour, sister or partner. Some open their bowels twice daily, others every 2–3 days. Many people come scurrying to their GP because they haven't 'gone' for three days. Often they forget to relate bowel waste evacuation with quantity of food consumed.

Also, bowels, like other organs, occasionally require a rest. This rest maybe needs a little gentle prompting if it persists, but by and large you're far healthier relaxing on the subject and allowing affairs to take their course.

Signs that you do need some help, include a bloated abdomen, having to strain, bad taste in your mouth and bad breath, a dull ache in the lower left abdomen, bad-smelling stools (due to putre-faction), and difficulty in losing weight. I will explain in Chapter 3, how to support your bowel and other detox organs, and offer them a helping hand (when needed).

So, you see, warning symptoms of toxin accumulation *do* develop but, since they're often vague and trivial, you may ignore them or blame them on age, overwork, even the weather! Most people are simply not attuned to what their bodies are trying to tell them. Toxin build-up has been linked to a variety of disorders and, wher-ever the blame lies, detoxing often brings relief.

Looking at toxins and common ailments

The most common toxin-linked ailments include:

- ✔ **Nervous system:** faintness, dizziness, headaches, migraines, pins and needles/other nerve pains, poor quality sleep, tiredness, lethargy, drowsiness, poor concentration, poor short-term memory. Migraine, for example, can be caused by personal sensitivity to certain foods, most notably oranges, peppermint, chocolate, garlic, and onions. Tiredness and poor sleep can be due to caffeine in tea and coffee.

- ✔ **Hangover symptoms:** headache, dizziness, raised body temperature, profuse sweating, extreme thirst, sleep disturbances, lethargy and fatigue, palpitations, racing pulse, restlessness, anxiety, agitation, tremor ('the shakes'), irritability, low mood, or recurrence of depression. The symptoms are due to the toxic breakdown products of alcohol, which accumulate in the bloodstream after a drinking binge as the liver strives to deal with them and the bowel and kidneys to excrete them.

- ✔ **Allergic conditions:** asthma, eczema, hay fever, urticaria (nettlerash or hives), itchy, inflamed eyes. Allergies and food sensitivities result from impairment to the immune defence system. This can be innate – that is, inherited – and/or triggered by an overload of toxins of many different varieties, such as artificial food additives and chemicals, if a sluggish bowel allows them to gather in the gut.

- ✔ **Appetite control/digestive system:** poor appetite, food cravings, binge eating, overweight or clinical obesity, difficulty in losing excess weight, food allergies/intolerances, nausea, burping, bad taste in mouth, 'dirty' coated tongue, wind, heartburn, acid reflux, bloated stomach, stomach ache, constipation, abdominal pain, *diverticulitis* (inflammation of tiny pouches in large bowel), irritable bowel syndrome, gall bladder inflammation, diarrhoea, constipation, offensive (foul-smelling) stools, mucus in stools, piles (haemorrhoids), raised blood fats and raised liver enzymes. Food cravings, binge eating, overweight and obesity are often linked to highs and lows of blood glucose level. Large quantities of refined sugar, needed nutritionally in small quantities, is generally responsible, under which circumstances it can be said to become a toxin. Most of the other symptoms are due to a sluggish bowel and chronic constipation.

✔ **Circulatory system:** flushes, excess sweating, a racing pulse, palpitations. Linked toxins can include caffeine as before, and refined sugar, which causes these symptoms when the blood glucose level falls below normal (hypoglycaemia).

✔ **Lungs and airways system:** frequent infections, heavy mucus production in nose and mouth, bad breath (halitosis), blocked sinuses, sore throat, recurrent dry cough, recurrent wet cough (with heavy mucus). Common causes of this are cigarette smoke and industrial fumes.

✔ **Muscular and skeletal system:** sore, aching joints; stiff, aching neck or back; early osteo- and rheumatoid arthritis; gout. Gout is due to a collection of uric acid, a toxic waste of your body's metabolism, in joints and nearby tissues. Faulty metabolism is often to blame, as are certain diuretic drugs such as bendroflumethiazide (a water pill prescribed for fluid retention and swollen ankles).

✔ **Reproductive and urinary system:** frequency of urination, scalding urine, strong and/or offensive urine, swollen ankles due to kidney malfunction, urinary infections, *urethritis* (inflammation of urethra, the bladder outlet tube), premenstrual syndrome, heavy or painful periods, difficulty in conceiving, low sperm count, low sex drive. Bad-smelling urine is most often due to an infection, for which you should see your GP. Other symptoms include frequent urination, passing small quantities of urine, getting up to urinate several times at night, and a scalding sensation on emptying your bladder. Strong urinary odours can also be caused by water-soluble toxins in the urine, such as the breakdown products of alcohol and artificial food additives, are excreted in urine, an offensive odour can sometimes be explained by this.

✔ **Skin complaints/complexion:** dry itchy skin, psoriasis, acne, pimples, boils, dark circles below eyes on waking, puffy eyelids. Puffiness may be due to water retention, and too much saturated fat and sugar are believed by some experts to help cause acne. Psoriasis is closely linked to high stress levels, a source of toxin attack on the immune system

Never assume that any symptoms persisting despite simple home remedies are caused by toxins (or anything else). Always see your doctor for a medical diagnosis and treatment.

Encountering Toxins Where They – and You – Live

Toxins come from the environment and also from inside your body. Environmental toxins range from airborne pollution due to living near a refuse disposal site or heavy road traffic, to bacterial toxins and artificial food additives that can be encountered in contaminated water supplies. Toxins from within your body include mercury from tooth fillings (for instance), and potentially-harmful food additives, which start as part of the environment and become internalised once you have digested the food in which they are carried.

Considering toxins without

Are environmental toxins *really* lurking round every corner, waiting to nab you? Don't a fresh home, hygienic kitchen surfaces, and safe food handling keep your home inviolate? You may even buy eco-friendly cleaning materials, keep household sprays to a minimum, and de-flea Felix and Fido with herbal dusting powders.

But do you also filter your drinking water? Do you wear a mask and protective clothing when putting insecticide on your plants? Do you check gas appliances for leaks, using a special kit? Avoid obsessing over unseen hazards – the stress only creates *more* free radicals to worry about! But it's still worthwhile to know about the toxins that you encounter in your daily contact with air, land, and water.

Wafting through the air

A huge number of toxins get pumped into the atmosphere although the ones that you most often read about are road-traffic emissions – the products of petrol and diesel fuel in automotive engines.

Getting the gas from carbon monoxide

You probably associate deadly carbon monoxide with reports of holiday tragedies – unsuspecting tourists warming up a chilly evening by switching on an innocent-looking gas heater, and dying from carbon monoxide poisoning. In fact, CO (the chemical notation for carbon monoxide) is also produced in undesirable amounts by cars and other motor engines, which between them account for 90 per cent of CO present in European urban areas. You'd never suspect that CO is around, though, as it's odourless, making it one toxin that really *can* creep up on you unawares.

Atmospheric CO levels may affect you if you have chronic bronchitis, emphysema or asthma because it reduces the blood's oxygen-carrying capacity. If you suffer from any of these conditions, your oxygen-carrying capacity is already lower than normal and atmospheric CO will only make things worse. Everyone inhales some atmospheric CO, and you're unlikely to be affected unless you have these lung conditions. All the same, CO does no one any good, and it's best to steer clear of avoidable sources like cigarette smoke where possible.

Avoid high-traffic areas wherever possible, especially if you have a chronic chest condition or if you're jogging. It's not healthy to breath heavily in an area full of car fumes! In your home, install a carbon-monoxide detector alarm and check gas heaters and stoves regularly.

Weighing the danger of lead

You may think of lead poisoning (if you think of it at all) as the relic of a bygone age. Didn't it go out with lead-based paints, and lead plumbing? While these two sources no longer pose a widespread threat (although industrial piping and paints can still contain the metal) lead and other heavy metals are still being ejected into the atmosphere as small particles during waste incineration, industrial metal processing, and fossil-fuel combustion.

Lead toxicity causes disorders of the central nervous system, mouth, gut, and other systems, and it affects brain function and personality development, especially in children, and is a major cause of infertility.

Remember the possibility of lead in old paint and pipe work when renovating an old property. Don't let children play with car batteries, suck metal objects, or put DIY paint or paintbrushes in their mouths.

Growing wary of agricultural and garden chemicals

You're probably aware of insecticides because you buy them for use in the home or garden, but you may also be brought into unconscious contact with them from unwashed fruit and vegetables and/or living in the country close to farmland, which is sprayed with chemicals. The following sections talk about the more common garden toxins you may come into contact with.

Avoiding aldicarb

Aldicarb is used in Britain for the cultivation of potatoes, carrots, parsnips, onions, ornamentals, and sugar beet (cattle feed). Aldicarb is brilliant at slaying eelworms and a variety of vegetable parasites and, as a bonus, kills off greenfly and other aphids, too.

Aldicarb is one of the most toxic pesticides ever manufactured. It plays havoc with wildlife and also causes convulsions, headaches, blurred vision, abnormal heart rhythm, diarrhoea, and vomiting in humans.

Be especially vigilant until 2007 when, following proposals by the European Commission, aldicarb will be finally and totally withdrawn from the marketplace. Also wash your hands regularly (and wear protective clothing) if you have to handle or operate machinery as a farmer or professional gardener in contact with aldicarb, or live close to farmland on which it is used.

Staying away from other pesticides

A recent study reported in the *New Scientist* on 26 May 2005, linked pesticide use with an increased risk of Parkinson's disease, a central nervous system disorder that affects 120,000 people in Britain and claims 10,000 new cases every year.

Pesticide toxins, which can be absorbed through the skin but generally enter the bloodstream after being inhaled, damage the central nervous system, giving rise to muscular stiffness, tremors, slow movements, poor co-ordination and balance, and other symptoms of Parkinson's disease.

Research shows that amateur gardeners, classed as having low pesticide exposure, have a 9 per cent increased risk of developing Parkinson's, while professional gardeners and farmers are 43 per cent more likely to suffer from it.

Follow the advice of Professor Anthony Seaton of Aberdeen University, who recommends that all pesticide users should wear masks and protective clothing to minimise exposure. Follow safety advice on packages, and check out eco-friendly alternatives to industrial chemicals.

Note: Food additives are a huge subject, requiring more than a paragraph or two under this section. Therefore, I address toxins found in food separately in Part II.

Household Water

British drinking water is generally, well . . . drinkable. Trips outside Europe may make you long for the tap water back home – chlorine and all! At least you can use it for drinking, showering, and teeth cleaning without the risk of dysentery. But should you be concerned about chlorine and other impurities in which water abounds? The short answer is yes; read on for the long answer.

Escaping chlorine

Chlorine is brilliant at killing off bugs and protecting you from killer diseases such as typhoid fever, dysentery, and cholera. (The withdrawal of chlorine from Peru's drinking water resulted in a cholera epidemic of 300,000 cases.) But chlorine also interacts with organic matter in water, forming dreadful-sounding substances called trihalomethanes, which can harm you. You would be most likely to encounter these compounds in inadequately treated drinking water supplies, in which the added chlorine could, and would, interact with, for instance, animal and human waste debris.

According to research at the Medical College of Wisconsin and Harvard University, chlorinated domestic water increases the risks of developing a range of cancers, especially of the bladder and rectum. We are talking here, not about the trihalomethanes but about chlorine itself, when it appears in water supplies in excessive amounts. And you're not only at risk if you swallow the stuff – it seems that your lungs and skin absorb nearly 100 times more chlorine and allied toxins during long, hot showers (and, to a lesser extent, baths) than you ever get from drinking tap water.

Use a filter jug for drinking water; or install an under-sink or whole-of-house water filter. You'll easily find companies that install this equipment on the Internet.

Leaving aluminium alone

You may have read about links between aluminium and Alzheimer's disease, which has been suspected for decades. Aluminium is generally thought to be one of a number of factors that collectively increase the risk of Alzheimer's.

In 1993, a report from the University of Manchester looked at whether the aluminium in domestic water (which is added during treatment processes) could be a contributing factor to Alzheimer's disease. Two points are worth noting:

- ✔ Although aluminium compounds become unstable and hyper-active when used to treat water, this activity doesn't actually increase your absorption of it. (The same applies to tea, a recognised source of body aluminium.)

- ✔ Household water supplies increase the amount of aluminium in your body. A study of children's teeth showed that the teeth of those living in areas where the aluminium content of water was high contained significantly larger amounts of this element than those living in low-aluminium water areas.

To reduce the amount of aluminium you take in, filter your water. It is also wise to avoid cooking with aluminium utensils, drinking from aluminium cans (except in an emergency), and using antiperspirants containing the metal.

Looking for toxins within

You have toxins inside you, right enough – and getting rid of them is what detoxing is all about. But if you drink alcohol moderately (or not at all), do not smoke, and try to eat healthily, where do you get these toxins from? The next sections explain the sources, some of which may surprise you.

Eliminating environmental toxins

Once environmental toxins enter your body, they become toxins within. How long they hang around making nuisances of themselves depends upon their tenacity, and your detox organs' abilities to boot them out.

Many water-soluble toxins such as caffeine, some food dyes, artificial sweeteners, and the products of alcohol breakdown are extracted from the blood by the kidneys and expelled in urine. Others, however, such as dioxins (which come from a variety of sources) are fat-soluble and, while the liver does a brilliant job in getting rid of many of them in bile, some get overlooked and are stored for months, or even years, in your body fat.

Internalising toxins in your body

These include:

Chewing over mercury amalgam dental fillings

Although mercury amalgam fillings (MAFs) initially come from outside your body, they become part of your body and can release toxins over many years. It is in fact calculated that around 40 per cent of the mercury in a MAF is released as an interior toxin within the first ten years of being in place. Mercury is a highly toxic element. Large quantities are linked to madness and even smaller amounts can damage the central nervous system.

An excess of mercury in your system can cause changes in the brain. Symptoms include irritability, mood swings, reduced concentration, short-term memory loss, lack of self-confidence, anxiety, low moods, poor quality sleep, and chronic tiredness. All of these symptoms are also features of clinical depression and one wonders how often MAFs have been passed over as a possible cause for the illness. Remember the Mad Hatter in *Alice in Wonderland?* Mercury used to be used in hat making!

Do not have MAFs inserted or removed while you are detoxing. After you detox, talk to your dentist about having MAFs removed and replaced with a non-toxic filling agent. It is calculated that your body takes a month for every year a MAF has been in place to get rid of all the mercury in your system.

You take a chelating agent as part of a detox (see Chapter 1 for the ingredients in a detox regimen). Chelating agents such as vitamin C, combine with toxic metals such as mercury, helping to neutralise the toxic metal's ill effects, and aid the body in its removal. Take further chelating agents while you're having MAFs removed.

Additional sources of mercury include industrial waste/landfill sites, fish – particularly tuna – from polluted waters, fungicides and other pesticides.

Investigating microbial toxins

Toxins within the body can also come from *microbes,* a blanket term for fungi, bacteria, viruses, and/or parasites. The substances they make when in your body can be especially irritating and toxic. To minimise suffering from their effects, you need to boost your immune defence system with regular detoxes (for example, twice yearly), and eat a wide range of fresh fruit and vegetables daily. You can supplement the antioxidant nutrients you obtain from plant foods by means of vitamin and mineral supplements. Reduce the risks of contracting vaginal thrush by taking antibiotics only when you have to, and seeing that your partner, if not circumcised, is also treated with an anti-fungal cream to prevent reinfection. Vaginal thrush can sometimes be cured by daily vaginal insertions of plain, live-culture yoghurt.

Thrashing a Candida (thrush) infection

Oral *Candida* infection causes unpleasant white plaques in the mouth. Vaginal thrush causes a thick, white, cheesy-smelling discharge and intense inflammation and itchiness. Both have toxic (that is, potentially injurious) properties, but intestinal thrush is most often associated with internal toxin production.

Due in part to the loss of friendly intestinal bugs – perhaps due to recent antibiotic courses – the *Candida* fungus can thrive within the gut. Many experts claim it causes symptoms ranging from ME (myalgic encephalomyelitis, also known as chronic fatigue syndrome), irritable bowel syndrome and diverticulitis flare-ups, to constipation and/or diarrhoea, abdominal bloating, and a chronically low mood.

Intestinal *Candida* may also help to explain certain food sensitivities and allergic reactions. The fungus multiplies by extending long tendrils called *hyphae* that penetrate the mucous membrane lining of the gut in search of nutriment. Capillaries become damaged, and fragments of hyphae seep into the bloodstream as do partially digested fluid and food particles. Both are interpreted (correctly) as foreign bodies by the immune system, which may then set up its defence mechanism of manufacturing antibodies to combat the invaders (thereby giving rise to allergic-type symptoms).

Beating bacteria

Pathogenic (disease causing) bacteria – both the organisms and the poisons that they secrete – constitute a huge group of widely varying toxins affecting everyone at times. Food poisoning is familiar to everyone: E. coli (a normal gut resident) and Salmonella (occasionally found in eggs) are common culprits and cause diarrhoea, sickness, stomach pains, and occasionally shock due to fluid loss and a particularly virulent toxin strain.

To reduce the risks of bacteria-borne disease, wash your hands after using the lavatory, rinse salad leaves as well as fruit and vegetables, and avoid commercially prepared food that may have been visited by flies. Cook raw food, such as meat, fish, poultry, and eggs thoroughly, and follow safety guidelines for food preparation and storage.

Steering clear of viruses

Viruses are another huge group of toxins that affect you in myriad ways. They're even more of a law unto themselves than bacteria which, although they can develop resistance to antibiotics, are easier to identify and treat. Common colds and flu, measles, mumps and chickenpox, shingles, laryngitis, viral pneumonia, viral meningitis, and glandular fever are all caused by virus toxins within.

Considering metabolic toxins

Metabolic toxins are substances your body produces as part of its normal function, or as a coping mechanism to deal with disease or injury. I consider both types in the following sections.

Producing your own, normal bodily by-products

This may sound like a fancy name for urine, sweat, and faeces, but I'm dealing here with by-products that tend to escape your notice, such as

 ✔ **Carbon dioxide** is a normal waste gas expelled continually by the lungs, but it can accumulate in your blood if you suffer from certain lung disorders. Chronic bronchitis and emphysema, severe chronic asthma, and some other disorders impair respiration so that too little oxygen is taken in by the lungs, and too little carbon dioxide given off. Once carbon dioxide is allowed to accumulate, it soon shows its nasty nature!

Your body deals with the surplus carbon dioxide that accumulates in this way, by forming larger than usual quantities of *carbonic acid* (which is just carbon dioxide dissolved in the blood or tissue). This acidifies the blood or, more correctly, renders it less alkaline. Your symptoms depend on the underlying illness, but in general, you can expect your condition to worsen and, if the condition is inadequately treated, you risk coma and death. As I said, carbon dioxide can be a *very* nasty toxin.

If you're prescribed oxygen for a chronic lung condition, ensure you take it according to instructions – even if the nasal tube or mask is an occasional nuisance.

✔ **Uric acid** is one toxin all gout sufferers have heard of! Uric acid is produced during the normal breakdown of your body cells as old cells are replaced by new ones and during digestion of plant and animal tissue. All food contains some uric acid. The chief waste product of protein digestion (from whatever source) is ammonia, which can also be a source of uric acid production.

The kidneys dispose of uric acid but, if it accumulates, uric acid appears as crystals around the joints, especially the joint at the base of the big toe. Typical gout symptoms develop, including burning, inflammation, and intense pain around affected joints. Repeated attacks can deform joints, and large deposits of uric acid, called *tophi,* may appear within the bones, or the skin of the ear.

Urate stones, made from this acid, can also form in the kidneys and interfere with the release of urine down the ureters to the bladder.

If you take thiazide diuretics such as benzoflurothiazide (mainly prescribed to treat high blood pressure), ask your doctor to check your uric acid blood levels from time to time. These drugs can raise uric acid levels above normal limits.

✔ **Cholesterol** is a word that may start you fretting over your personal blood level. Actually, cholesterol is an essential metabolic player, and, like carbon dioxide, only acts as a toxin when too much is present, and/or in the wrong place.

Your body makes cholesterol from which it manufactures sex and adrenal gland hormones, bile salts, and other compounds. The rest comes from diet – fatty meat, butter, cream, and other sources of saturated fat. LDL cholesterol (the low density lipoprotein or bad variety) tends to form deposits within the walls of arteries, leading to a clogged blood supply, heart attack, and stroke.

But even some toxins boast devil and angel faces! The dangerous action of LDLs are opposed by those of the healthy variety – known as HDL or high density lipoprotein cholesterol.

Cut down on saturated animal fats and substitute cold-pressed vegetable oils and their products, which are high in healthy omega-rich polyunsaturates, to maximise your healthy cholesterol.

Protecting yourself with by-products

Your body produces thousands of helpful substances using a vast range of mechanisms, all designed to keep your systems balanced and working harmoniously. Sometimes it makes a mistake, though, as in the case of allergies and the production of auto-antibodies. Pus formation is also a protective mechanism against encroaching harmful bacteria, although its appearance generally gives rise to alarm.

- **Antibodies:** Nothing like your average toxin, by any means, antibodies nevertheless can have a highly damaging effect if your immune defence system manufactures them by mistake. The real purpose of these complex protein molecules is to bind with and incapacitate true bodily threats such as germs and foreign bodies. But problems arise when the immune system misidentifies harmless substances such as pollen, antibiotics, or strawberries (for instance) as threatening. Subsequent encounters with these substances release a whole army of antibodies specifically geared to react with them, and rashes, wheezing, faintness, vomiting, and/or other allergic symptoms develop.

  Another example of antibodies behaving as toxins is the group known as autoantibodies, seen in people with so-called autoimmune diseases such as lupus (Lupus erythematosis), rheumatoid arthritis, ulcerative colitis, and Crohn's disease, which affects the small intestine. In all of these, the immune cells react to the body's own tissue as though it were a foreign substance. Extensive, debilitating inflammation can, if not adequately treated, wreak severe joint and organ damage, showing the toxin-like nature of misapplied antibodies.

- **Pus:** Have you ever thought of pus as a toxin? It is one, right enough – you'll doubtless have noticed how easy it is to infect a clean cut or graze with pus from an infected wound. The swift spread of *impetigo* (school sores) from one child to many others with whom they're in contact is just one example.

Pus is a mixture of white blood cells that engulf and destroy invading organisms, together with a few red cells, lots of dead and dying bacteria such as *Pseudomonas, Streptococcus,* and *Staphylococcus,* and fragments of dead tissue. It's produced by inflammation, one of the most important defence mechanisms protecting you from being overcome by dangerous invading organisms.

Chapter 3

Supporting Your Detox Organs

*Y*our body gets rid of toxins through your liver, kidneys, gut, skin, and lungs. You're doubtless aware of the need for a healthy skin, but may not have considered its toxin-zapping actions nor those of your other four 'invisible' eliminatory organs.

In this chapter, I tell you how to keep these vital organs happy and well-functioning during detox.

Looking After Your Liver

Your liver is a large, red-brown glandular organ. The liver carries out many important functions, such as making bile, changing food into energy, and cleaning alcohol and poisons from the blood. It also makes vitamin A.

Few people give their liver a passing thought so it's just as well that the liver is a forgiving organ. Although it's exposed to toxins every millisecond of every single day, the liver's great powers of regeneration enable it to struggle on regardless. Without your liver toxins would overwhelm your body, and you would feel, and become, very unwell. Treat your mate with respect!

Like most good mates, your liver is tolerant, forgiving, and unbelievably obliging. Even if surgeons removed 90 per cent of it, the remaining 10 per cent would do its best to grow back!

However, your liver often needs extra support. Just caring for your liver brings detox benefits and allows you to say 'I'm detoxing'.

Getting the low-down on your liver

The liver doesn't just peep coyly from a dinner plate flanked by onions and bacon. It holds court in the upper right-hand quarter of your abdomen, protected by your ribs and overhanging your stomach and pancreas. It consists of a left and a right lobe, each containing billions of liver cells *(hepatocytes)* arranged in six-sided columns or lobules. Oxygen, nutrients, and toxins reach these liver cells through spaces called *sinusoids* found throughout the liver.

 Your liver is your body's largest gland, weighing around 1.4 kilograms. The peculiar thing about the liver is that it has a double blood supply. The hepatic artery brings it oxygen-rich blood to stoke your liver's fires, while the hepatic portal vein brings it all the nutrients, goodies and baddies including toxins absorbed from your stomach and gut.

Most detoxifying processes start in the liver, which has more detox enzymes than any other organ. It certainly needs them – the hepatic portal vein carries huge numbers of toxins daily to your liver from your bowel.

Your liver helps keep your body clean by

- ✔ Making bile to digest fatty foods in the small bowel (see the next section for an explanation of bile)
- ✔ Storing carbohydrate as a source of energy fuel
- ✔ Producing glucose to maintain your blood sugar level.

 Glucose is the main type of sugar in the blood and is the major source of energy for the body's cells. Glucose comes from the foods you eat and the body can make it from other substances. Glucose is carried to the cells through the bloodstream. Several hormones, including insulin, control glucose levels in the blood by

- ✔ Forming vital substances such as albumin and globulin, the proteins present in the bloodstream that aid cell activity and manufacture antibodies; and blood-clotting agents

✔ Making cholesterol, which is used by the body to manufacture healthy cell walls and many hormones and other body chemicals, and triglycerides – a form of storage for fat in the bloodstream

✔ Producing *urea,* a waste nitrogen product removed in urine.

Bringing up bile, as in bilious

Your liver's most useful agent is bile, that bitter substance you've probably brought up during a bilious attack or stomach upset. *Bile* is a greenish-yellow liquid containing organic acids, salts, pigments, and other chemicals. Your liver makes around 400 to 800 millilitres daily.

Bile is stored and concentrated in the gall bladder until you eat. The digestive process triggers the release of bile into the duodenum (the first section of the small intestine). If you've had your gall bladder removed, bile trickles straight into your duodenum without being stored. Bile *emulsifies* dietary fats, meaning it breaks them down into small particles to make them easier to digest. Bile also acts as a storage area to collect and transport toxins, cholesterol, and waste substances from your liver into your intestines for voiding.

Bile is potent stuff – and very valuable to the body. Around 95 per cent of the amount you make is reabsorbed and recycled back to the liver. In fact, you reuse each bile salt molecule around 20 times – sometimes up to three times just while digesting a single meal.

Examining the inner workings

Your liver is a real workaholic, beavering away round the clock to clear toxins before they can make you ill. The liver has three methods of getting rid of toxins. It can

✔ Chemically alter toxins into (generally) less toxic, more water-soluble compounds that can be removed in urine, sweat, intestinal juices, and tears

✔ Secrete them into bile so that the toxins pass out through your intestines

✔ Surround and digest toxins as well as bacteria and viruses.

The liver uses a neat, two-step process to handle some toxins, for instance alcohol:

1. **Using the first of the three methods mentioned above, the liver cells convert the miscreant toxin (A) into substance (B), which may be more poisonous than A.**

For example, when you drink wine or beer, the liver breaks down the innocent-tasting alcohol (A) into horrible acetaldehyde (B).

2. **The cells quickly join (or *conjugate*) (B) with a helpful carrier molecule such as glucuronate or glutathione to become compound (C), which is a good deal safer and far easier to dispose of than the original toxin (A).**

Acetaldehyde is then converted into good old acetate (C), which your body can safely burn releasing energy, carbon dioxide, and water.

Interestingly, when your liver is exposed to lots of the same toxin it manufactures more of the enzymes needed to process it. Regular heavy drinkers, for instance, have higher than normal levels of alcohol-detoxing enzymes. These can show up on a routine blood test, even if you haven't touched a drop for days.

The good news is that these enzymes clear the relevant toxins more efficiently than normal when you start a detox. Giving up alcohol or reverting to lower, safer drinking levels can return the enzyme levels to normal.

Over-exposure to toxins can make your liver sluggish, however, causing bloating, fullness, wind, nausea, and general feelings of *yuk!* Don't blame your liver unnecessarily, however, as simply overeating or drinking can cause the same symptoms.

Helping your liver

The first phase of detoxification is carried out by the cytochrome P450 series of enzymes, which you may have heard of because they are important in processing many prescribed drugs. These generate free radicals during their action, so a good intake of antioxidants is vital, especially during detox. Cytochrome P450 reactions also need good supplies of certain vitamins and minerals to work properly.

Drinking too much grapefruit juice can slow the action of first phase detox. This is why you mustn't consume this fruit or its juice when detoxing or taking certain prescribed and over-the-counter drugs.

The herbal remedies and dietary supplements I discuss in the following sections can lighten your liver's workload.

Probiotics also play an important role in liver health but are mainly associated with the digestive tract, so I discuss them in the 'Encouraging bacteria' section later in this chapter.

Avoiding alcohol for liver health

If you drink too rapidly, or too much, your liver can accumulate a backlog of work and/or become short of conjugating materials. An intoxicated liver can allow super-toxic acetaldehyde to build up, causing the dreaded hangover symptoms.

Heavy drinking can cause liver damage, in particular ghastly-sounding conditions like fatty degeneration, hepatitis (inflammation), and liver cell death. Within the liver, poorly functioning patches of struggling liver cells become mixed up at random with scar tissue, which forms where the cells die. The healthy cells continue multiplying, bless 'em, creating nodules squashed by scar tissue which nips and depletes their blood supply. The liver becomes shrunken and knobbly and cannot deal with its normal workload, a condition known as alcoholic cirrhosis. This can progress for a while without causing symptoms, so may be quite advanced by the time you start to feel the effects. If you carry on drinking heavily, you will eventually need a liver transplant. Looking on the bright side, fatty liver cells poisoned by excess alcohol are often able to repair themselves if you stop drinking.

Mopping up milk thistle (silybum marianum)

Milk thistle grows on dry, rocky wasteland in southern and western Europe and in North America.

Active ingredients include bioflavonoids, useful plant chemicals with strong antioxidant properties. A prime one in milk thistle is silymarin, which has at least 200 times the antioxidant oomph of vitamin C. Many studies show that silymarin helps protect liver cells from attacks by alcohol, medical chemotherapy, and even death-cap mushrooms.

Silvmarin's actions include:

- ✔ Mopping up free radicals, which are hyperactive oxygen mole-cules that harm the immune system when present in excessive numbers. Triggers to their production in the body include stress, smoking, ageing, cancer, viral illnesses, sunlight, and other forms of radiation. Mopping them up, that is putting them out of action, reduces their noxious effects and helps to protect the immune system.

- ✔ Boosting levels of glutathione, the liver's own super-oxidant

- ✔ Reinforcing liver cell membranes to slow down entry of over-loads of toxins

- ✔ Reducing scar tissue formation

> ✔ Aiding liver cell regeneration
>
> ✔ Stimulating bile secretion.

Milk thistle can be a useful tonic if you drink alcohol regularly or lead a toxic, 21st-century lifestyle. It is sold in capsule form by pharmacists and health food shops. Take 70 mg twice daily between meals for a tonic for three weeks at a time twice yearly between detoxes. A typical detox dose is 100 mg thrice daily, increasing by 50 mg daily every three days until you reach a maximum of 200 mg thrice daily. Your liver function can start to pick up within as little as five days.

Milk thistle has few reported side effects. The commonest is a mild laxative effect. If you suffer from gallstones or liver disease, take milk thistle only under the guidance of a medical doctor or qualified medical herbalist.

Digging dandelion

Dandelion *(Taraxacum officinalis)* may be a pest to keen gardeners, but its leaves in spring have been prized for centuries as a herbal tonic, and its roots (especially from two-year-old plants) have beneficial all-round detoxifying properties. Dandelion aids liver cleansing by stimulating its detox functions and bile flow (and thereby the elimination of toxic waste by the intestines).

Add fresh young dandelion leaves or freshly sliced root to salads – pick from unpolluted sites only. Try boiling the leaves and eating them like spinach. If you use chemical controls in your garden then don't use any dandelions that survive the treatment as they will be polluted with the chemicals.

Take 5 to 10 g fresh root daily in two equal doses (2-year-old plants are recommended), or a 500 mg extract twice daily. Dandelion is sold by pharmacists and health food stores.

If you have gallstones, take dandelion only under qualified medical or herbal supervision. Avoid taking dandelion during an acute gallstones attack (known medically as cholecystitis) and other forms of obstructive jaundice.

Gaining from gotu kola

Gotu kola *(Centella asiatica)*, a small herb with umbrella-shaped leaves found in the tropical Near and Far East, is claimed to extend human lifespan. Legend has it that it helped the Chinese herbalist LiChing Yun live for 256 years!

Widely used in Ayurvedic (traditional Indian) medicine where it is called a *brahmi,* gotu kola aids detox by cleansing the blood and the liver, and improves the health of liver cells in people with cirrhosis.

Despite its name, gotu kola is unrelated to the kola nut (or cola nut) and contains no caffeine.

Take three capsules standardised to contain 2½ mg of triterpenes (this plant's active ingredients) per capsule daily.

If the dose mentioned gives you a headache, try halving it (the dose, not the capsule), as even a half dose will bring benefits. If headaches persist, stop taking it.

Turmeric

Everyone warns you against takeaways, but some of the ingredients in ethnic dishes have powerful medicinal properties. Turmeric (Curcuma longa) is widely used in Indian cookery to flavour and colour rice and other dishes, and has been used for many centuries in Ayurvedic and traditional Chinese medicine to cleanse the liver.

Turmuric's active ingredient, curcumin, is a potent anti-inflammatory antioxidant that stimulates bile secretion and the production of two liver detox enzymes – glutathione-s-transferase and glucuronyl transferase. Curcumin also encourages the regeneration of liver cells, reduces blood clotting, and helps to lower raised cholesterol.

Try two level teaspoonfuls of turmeric powder mixed into juices, soups, stews, or what have you twice daily when detoxing.

Being sure to get your vitamin B complex

Perhaps you've heard of vitamin B6 (pyridoxine), which relieves premenstrual tension (PMT) and carpal tunnel syndrome, or thiamine (B1), which features in the standard treatment regimen of alcohol detox units.

Liver cells need B complex vitamins for energy production and to help process alcohol and other toxins. Collectively, B complex vitamins release energy during the metabolic breakdown of fats, carbohydrates and proteins, and are vital to the liver, which depends upon on-going supplies of energy.

Stress and a high alcohol intake both deplete water-soluble B complex vitamin stores so, in one way or another, most of us need B complex supplements.

When 150 viral hepatitis sufferers took B5 (pantothenic acid) supplements, their liver function tests improved significantly, and they made more antibodies, fighting the infection more effectively. Pantothenic acid apparently has a protective effect on liver cells even when overwhelmed by viral toxins.

Try taking a vitamin B complex supplement with a combined dose of 50 mg. If you drink a lot of alcohol, you may need 100 mg B complex. These supplements are often referred to as Vitamin B 50 complex or Vitamin B 100 complex.

Mooning about selenium

A mineral named after the Greek Moon Goddess, Selene, selenium is obtained from plants that have grown on selenium-rich soils. You are unlikely to find such plants in Europe because most selenium leached out of the soil during the last Ice Age, although some sites exist in Germany and Italy where selenium occurs. Notable occurrences of minerals containing selenium are found in the Americas.

Selenium-containing amino acids form part of more than 20 important antioxidant enzymes, including the liver enzyme glutathione peroxidase, responsible for quenching harmful reactions sparked by ongoing toxin processing. Selenium also enhances the activities of the enzyme P450, and helps to repair damaged genetic material. Enzyme P450 helps to break down medication drugs so that they act beneficially but are excreted safely and not allowed to accumulate.

Selenium helps to protect you from liver cancer sparked by the huge toxic overload with which it deals.

Take 100 mcg (microgram) of selenium daily during detox. Consider doing so for life.

You can safely take up to 450 mcg of selenium daily but toxicity can occur above 800 mcg daily. Selenium toxicity signs include a garlicky body odour, blackened or fragile fingernails, a metallic taste in the mouth, nausea, dizziness, and hair loss.

Taking Care of Your Kidneys

Few people are aware of their kidneys until they suffer from a kidney ailment such as cystitis in which bugs climb the urinary tract to infect the kidneys, producing back pain and fever. Like your liver, however, your kidneys work best when understood and loved.

Your kidneys are expert jugglers: They balance and synchronise fluid and salt levels; excrete toxins; regulate blood pressure, red cell production, and blood and tissue pH. So respect them!

Keeping pace with your kidneys

Kidneys do far more than grace old-fashioned breakfast menus and make tasty pet food – they regulate your fluid and salt balance, for one thing, and dispose of oceans of nasty toxins.

Your kidneys are two bean-shaped organs on either side of your spine within the abdominal cavity, protected from behind by your back muscles and lower ribs. Each kidney wears a small pointy cap – the adrenal gland – and receives its own branch from the aorta and inferior vena cava (the body's principal artery and vein), which run between them.

Kidneys are the terrible twins – upset one (with diabetes, high blood pressure, an infection, for instance) and the other comes out in sympathy. You can manage very well with just one kidney and you can carry on quite happily with a pair of quite badly diseased ones before producing any symptoms. But *some* healthy kidney tissue is essential to life and health. To understand what the kidneys do – and how they do it – you need to know a little about their structure.

Observing the workings

Kidneys may not look all that clever, but they're actually hives of industry. Between them they contain around two million working units or nephrons, each of which starts as a minute twig (arteriole) of the renal artery. The arteriole forms a tangle of even tinier capillary vessels called the glomerular tuft, which is far more complicated than Spaghetti Junction. Each tuft is enclosed in a membranous bag or Bowman's capsule, which collects the watery solution filtered by the tuft from the blood. This solution drains into a narrow, winding renal tubule (the final part of the nephron) where it is condensed to a smaller amount of urine. The urine trickles into one of the many collecting tubules carrying urine to the renal pelvis.

Urine formed by the kidneys enters a funnel-shaped hollow, the renal pelvis, which narrows at the kidneys' inner margins (hilum) to form the ureter. This tube passes straight down the back of the abdomen for about 25 centimetres to the bladder. The renal artery carries blood from the aorta to the kidney and, once it has circulated, the renal vein returns it to the vena cava.

Finding out the functions

The first part of the nephron filters the blood, which enters it under high pressure from the renal artery. In doing so, it holds back blood cells and large protein molecules but allows water, salts, nutrients, and waste products to pass out of the glomerular tuft into the Bowman's capsule (where – surprise, surprise! – the fluid is known as the glomerular filtrate). The kidneys create around 120 millilitres (ml) per minute of this fluid, around 119 ml of which are reabsorbed in the final section of the nephron (part of the kidney) before its contents reach the renal pelvis, together with glucose, amino acid, and other nutrients.

Toxins and other waste products generally remain in the tubules to be excreted in the urine.

The kidneys work together with *aldosterone,* a hormone secreted by the adrenal glands, to keep the body's sodium levels within normal limits. Your kidneys retain sodium if you've lost a lot in sweat, for example, but if you take too much on board from salty food, or by accidentally swallowing seawater, they expel the excess in the urine.

The kidneys also

- ✔ Help to regulate the acidity of the body fluids, the balance of body fluids, and blood pressure
- ✔ Pump excess sodium from the blood into the urine while reabsorbing potassium – a vital mineral for all healthy cells
- ✔ Produce a hormone, erythropoietin, which controls the rate at which red blood cells are made in the bone marrow.

Fluid loss increases the dilution of the blood, prompting the brain's pituitary gland to release anti-diuretic hormone (ADH). ADH encourages the kidneys to reabsorb and conserve water, reducing the urine output.

Keeping acid at bay

You hear a lot about acidic and alkaline foods in connection with detox. The body's acidity/alkalinity is measured in pH, a scale running from highly acid (1) through neutral (7) to highly alkaline (14). A body's normal pH is 7.4, or slightly alkaline, and, because many by-products of body chemistry are acidic, you and your body have to make a constant effort to keep the pH at an acceptable level.

Because getting rid of acids is so vital, the kidneys have other means at their disposal besides excreting acid urine. They form ammonia, which neutralises acids to form ammonium salts, and they also take in alkaline phosphate from the blood but excrete acid phosphate in the urine (the phosphate essentially taking up the excess acid).

Under normal conditions, you pass about 1½ litres of urine daily. Although this amount can be increased to get rid of any likely excess of water, it cannot be safely reduced to less than 600 ml. This is the minimum amount of fluid needed to carry away waste toxins, and you have to drink this amount (plus enough to cover fluid loss from the gut, lungs, and skin) to stay alive and well.

If you're shipwrecked on a desert island – don't drink the seawater! When your body is short of salt, hardly any is excreted in the urine, but if salt is in excess, the urine's concentration of salt can reach two per cent. Seawater averages three per cent, so if you drink a pint of it you have to pass a pint and a half of urine to get rid of the salt. So, you run a greater risk of death by dehydration than if you drank nothing at all.

Backing your kidneys

Water, herbal remedies, and dietary supplements can nurture your kidneys and help them to deal with their heavy workload. In the following sections, I tell you how.

Drinking plain water

Water is essential to the body, especially when you are detoxin. You need to choose between the various forms available, but – whatever your choice – you should never, *but never*, forget to drink it. Drinking six to eight 250 ml glasses of water every day helps your kidneys in their regular tasks of balancing body fluids and pH, regulating salt levels and excreting toxins and waste. It also reduces the risks of developing kidney stones.

The choice of water is yours. The various mineral waters all have their fans, as does plain tap water – preferably filtered to remove bacteria, chlorine, and other impurities using a filtering jug or tap attachment. Some nutritionists suggest that room temperature still water is always the best choice, but I think this is a counsel of perfection. The important thing is to drink a litre to a litre and a half day-in and day-out – and if you prefer it chilled and sparkling, then go for it.

Just bear in mind that too much 'fizz' can cause unattractive burping and bloating, and has been blamed for causing cellulite (but then, what hasn't?) You should also avoid taking icy water after energetic exercise if you're keen to burn as many calories as possible (cold water can slow the metabolic rate of food fuel consumption).

If you have a glass of your water of choice on waking, a glass or two after each meal, and another glass or so between meals, you should find it easy to take in the required amount.

Taking the holiday out of cranberries

Juice of the cranberry *(Vaccinium macrocarpon)* reduces the risks of urinary tract infection by acidifying the urine and making it harder for bacteria to stick to the bladder's lining membrane. If you're prone to cystitis (bladder inflammation, usually, although not invariably, due to infection), daily or at least regular cranberry juice can help to reduce the frequency and severity of attacks. An untreated urine infection can ascend the ureters and reach the kidneys, turning a comparatively minor ailment into a more serious one.

While cranberry sauce goes with Christmas turkey, fresh cranberries are now widely available in supermarkets for most of the year. You can also juice these ripe berries in preference to buying commercial cranberry juice drinks loaded with sugar. Alternatively you can take cranberry capsules; just follow the instructions on the label. (Cranberry juice actually protects the whole of the urinary tract (from bladder up to the kidney's inner hollow or renal pelvis) from bacterial infection.)

No recommended amount of cranberry juice exists with regard to healthy kidneys, but try a glass daily and drink may be two or even three glasses daily during detox depending upon how much you like it! Canned or packaged cranberry juice is significantly diluted with water. You may like to add some water to freshly-squeezed cranberry juice.

Cranberries also supply a range of cancer-beating phytochemicals (plant substances); vitamins A, B complex, C, and E; and the minerals potassium, calcium, magnesium, iron, zinc, and phosphorus.

Cottoning on to corn silk

Corn silk is the beautifully descriptive name of the tassels you find when you peel open a cob of sweet corn. Even its botanical name, (Zea mays), sounds like a corn goddess!

Corn silk's diuretic action flushes out the urinary tract and encourages the healthy function of kidneys, bladder, and small bowel. It is also used to treat prostate gland disorders (which hamper urine flow), fluid retention due to premenstrual tension , and, interestingly, bed-wetting when taken several hours before bedtime. Used together with other 'kidney herbs', corn silk opens and cleans out the urinary tract and removes mucus from the bladder.

You can find corn silk in various herbal remedies for fluid retention and a healthy urinary tract. Take according to label instructions.

Doubling the benefits of dandelion

The dandelion's diuretic action improves kidney function and fluid retention. Dandelions, both the leaves and the root, also supply a range of minerals including potassium (many pharmaceutical diuretics cause a loss of potassium in the urine), calcium, iron, magnesium, and zinc; and vitamins C and B1, B2, and B3. Check out the 'Digging dandelion' section earlier in this chapter for additional benefits and tips.

Medical herbalists recommend 4–10 g of the dried leaf equivalent three times daily, during detox, and you can safely take this dose at three- to four- week intervals if you choose to (when not detoxing), say three times a year; or half this amount as a daily supplement, which you can find in chemists and health food stores.

Do not take dandelion in combination with prescription diuretics, nor if you suffer from gallstones or any obstruction of the biliary tract.

Softening up to marshmallow

Marshmallow *(Althaea officinalis)* helps to cleanse the kidneys and aids the expulsion of excess fluid and mucus from the urinary tract. Related to the hollyhock, marshmallow's safe, soothing properties make it a useful filler in the compounding of herbal pills. Marshmallow flowers are an ingredient in many herbal teas, and the plant as a whole – flowers, leaves, and roots – supplies a range of phytochemicals including beta carotene (provitamin A). Nutrients include vitamins B1, B2, B3, and C; amino acids; and the minerals zinc, calcium, magnesium, iron, phosphorus, and selenium.

Sip a cup of marshmallow tea daily when you're feeling bloated, or your bladder or kidneys are recovering from a urinary infection. Use the freshly picked or dried flowers, or take marshmallow as a herbal supplement, according to the manufacturer's instructions. There is no real difference between a detox and 'everyday' dose.

Touching On Skin

The skin's detox activities are most obvious when whiteheads, pimples, and other pus-filled spots appear, ready to discharge a load of toxins. However, a clear complexion shows few signs of the skin's hard work as a toxin-expeller.

Most people tend to concentrate skincare on the areas most on show. However, every part of your approximately 2½ square metres of skin has an important function, mostly elimination. Skin deserves all-over care, respect and regular help.

The skin's outer epidermis provides a tough, waterproof covering with an outer layer of dry, flattened dead cells. Replacements, which arrive as newly formed cells, push up from the underlying germinal layer. Below this layer lies the *dermis* (Latin for skin) consisting of a tough, elastic connective tissue containing blood vessels and nerves. Your sweat glands lie deep in the dermis and open onto the skin. Hair and nails develop from the epidermis – hair follicles (roots) also give rise to sebaceous (grease) glands, and nails develop as hard, tough sheets of keratin protein produced by cells in the base and sides of each nail.

How your skin works

Your skin eliminates poisons by

- Shedding toxins in sloughed-off dead cells
- Sweating away water-soluble toxins
- Excreting fat-soluble toxins in skin grease (sebum)
- Pushing out some toxins, including lead and other metals, in your nails and hair.

Other vital reasons why you and your skin are lifetime partners include all of the following:

- Provides a waterproof barrier (without it, you'd *really* know about water retention!)
- Guards delicate organs and tissues against infection and injury
- Helps to regulate body temperature
- Manufactures vitamin D with the aid of sunlight.

Skin cells soon become dehydrated if you fail to replace what they lose. Remember that increased urine output due to alcohol or caffeine-loaded drinks or water pills (diuretics) needs to be balanced by your daily water intake. Fortunately your skin cells are more than happy to take in water again when you offer them a drink! Skin cells are a bit like cuttings from a Busy Lizzie plant, whose large, fluid-filled cells soon lose colour and shape if they're deprived of water. Refresh them, and they plump out and grow as before. You're forgiven!

You lose fluid in obvious (and less obvious) ways. You know that you're losing fluid when you perspire heavily in hot weather or during vigorous exercise. Thirst makes you drink to replace the lost water (and hopefully salts). But do you think about replacing fluids when you suffer from diarrhoea and vomiting? In fact, dehydration is the chief cause of that washed-out feeling you have after an attack has subsided. Then there's the skin-drying effect of central heating and air conditioning, not to mention cold winter weather and high winds.

Hydration – continually replacing lost water – is essential to your skin's overall health and its detoxifying actions. But you can get so used to a chronic 'water shortage' that you fail to identify it. Instead, you suffer from headaches, tiredness, poor concentration, a bad taste in your mouth, bad breath, thick, sticky mucus, and – you've guessed it – dull, lifeless skin.

Soothing your skin

The following sections fill you in on some of the ways you can help your skin eliminate toxins.

Sweating it out

Exercise, saunas, steam treatments, and 'sweaty foods' all promote perspiration. Sweating is particularly helpful during the cleansing phase, as it helps to mobilise and release toxins stored in the fat layer under the skin.

You're better off avoiding strenuous exercise when following a juice and fruit diet – although it should be safe enough to get a little hot and sweaty using brisk walking or cycling on the flat. Once you are eating a full, healthy diet, you can exercise more vigorously according to your health and needs.

Other sweat-inducing methods include

- ✔ **Saunas:** Drink plenty of fluid during the sauna and stay only as long as you feel comfortable – everyone has a different tolerance of steamy, high temperatures.

  Try to take saunas a day or so before starting a detox programme because the hot, steamy conditions can make you feel faint. Alternatively, you can postpone a sauna until your main programme is complete, and you're eating a broad-based, healthy diet.

- ✔ **Steam treatments:** Steam just your face, using the head-over-towel method and a bowl of steaming water, or use a walk-in steam cabinet in a gym or salon.

- ✔ **Sweaty foods:** Hot vindaloo curries are notorious for causing their devotees to sweat! Chilli peppers also bring about healthy sweating and can be used fresh in recipes such as stir-fries, salads, and rice dishes, or added as a dried or powdered spice to any of these. Chilli has wide appeal and is now even present in certain chocolate bars to add variety and interest.

Treating with Dead Sea salts

These mineral salts and mud encourage the elimination of toxins and soothe conditions such as psoriasis and eczema, typified by inflammation and a shedding of dead surface cells. Warm mineral mud wraps are believed to combat cellulite and fluid retention.

Cosmetically, they give the skin new life and elasticity, and tighten any slackness. The skin acquires a glow and feels healthier and more comfortable. Use mud masks for your face – the mineral salts are too harsh.

Applying evening primrose oil

This plant seed extract is a rich source of the omega-6 nutrient gammalinolenic acid, which your body can manufacture from the cis-linoleic acid found in cold-pressed vegetable oils such as rape-seed and safflower. Factors such as ageing, viruses, unhealthy trans-fats in junk food, and UV rays can interfere with this process, leaving you short of hormone-like prostaglandins needed for the minute-by-minute control of skin cells and other bodily systems.

Clinical studies confirm the usefulness of evening primrose oil (EPO), rich in omega-6 GLA (gammalinolenic acid), in the treatment of eczema, and it's included in the formulations of numerous hair- and skin-care products.

EPO is known to enhance the health and vitality of skin, hair, and nails, and you can take it as a daily supplement (try two to three 500 mg capsules daily). Alternatively, soften the capsules in a little warm water and apply the contents directly to dry, roughened, and inflamed skin.

Getting a Lung-full

If you're keen on sports, or suffer from asthma, emphysema, or chronic bronchitis, then you'll be very aware of your lungs' importance. For most of us, though, it's more a case of 'out of sight, out of mind'. All the same, your life depends upon a continuous supply of oxygen and removal of waste, including carbon dioxide, water, and a range of inhaled toxins.

Outstripping the comedones

Blackheads (comedones) are plugs of skin grease lodged in the opening of a skin gland, preventing the normal discharge of sebum and fat-soluble toxins. The blackness is due to the grime their surfaces attract.

They can be difficult to remove, but you can try the following method. Ring out a face flannel in very hot water containing a drop or two of Tea Tree essential oil. Apply to the blackhead area. Then dry the skin and push gently inwards with the sides of your forefingers (not nails which should however, be short and clean).

When the blackhead emerges, it leaves a large, round, empty pore where the gland opening has become stretched. Splash regularly with cold water plus a little Tea Tree oil to encourage closure.

Being aware that lungs aren't just bellows

The lungs are as essential to life as your heart, liver, and brain, yet they're fairly passive players as far as breathing movements are concerned.

When you breathe in, your lungs do not expand by pushing out your chest wall. To breathe in you actually lower your *diaphragm* – the thick, powerful muscle sheet separating your chest (thorax) from your abdomen – aided and abetted by the muscles of your chest wall. As the hollow within your chest enlarges, negative pressure develops, causing the lungs to expand and fill the chest cavity. This draws in air through the nose and mouth and down the windpipe or trachea, which itself ends in a right and left branch (bronchus) each supplying a lung.

Within the lung, the bronchi branch into finer and finer twigs, eventually forming the tiniest twiglets of all, the bronchioles. In this way, air entering at the top of the respiratory tract eventually reaches the millions of minute, fragile air sacs (alveoli) appearing at the end of the smallest bronchioles.

The surface area of all the alveoli combined adds up to a staggering 180 square metres of respiratory membrane which is richly supplied with capillary blood vessels. This is where the oxygen that has been inhaled in air enters the bloodstream and carbon dioxide and other toxins such as acetone leave it to be released from the body as you breathe out.

Respecting the breath of life

Air clearly deserves this name since our lives depend on it. But the 'breath of life' is also a term for the life force, life energy or Chi – the element claimed to be present in all living things and absent from non-living ones. Known as 'ruah' in Hebrew, 'mana' in Polynesian, 'pneuma' in Greek and 'prana' to Yogis, the 'breath of life' is believed to be the healing element transmitted to patients during so-called miraculous cures.

Further, many wonderful, if unfathomable, properties are attributed to this force: Tibetan mystics are said to use secret breathing techniques to achieve *tumo* – the ability to remain healthily warm at sub-zero temperatures. Utilisation of prana, or breath of life, is also said to explain the performance of Indian siddhas such as mystical levitation and invisibility.

You don't have to meditate naked in the snow or discover how to fly to enjoy the stress-relieving benefits of healthy breathing. The exercise here can prevent typical stress respiration – quick, shallow, and irregular breaths that allow carbon dioxide to accumulate in the blood, thereby lowering your blood's pH, making it too acidic. Typical symptoms include a fluttery sensation in the chest, nausea, dizziness, pins and needles especially around your mouth, and sometimes panic attacks. To prevent such symptoms:

- Sit comfortably in your chair, circle your arms around at the shoulder joints, and hunch your shoulders a few times to dispel muscular tension.

- Breathe in through your mouth or mouth and nose (whichever feels more comfortable), expanding your chest and filling your lungs as fully as possible.

- Breathe in and out deeply, noticing the rise and fall of your abdomen rather than your chest – do this a total of six times.

- Go on breathing regularly to a count of three as you breathe in, and a count of four as you breathe out.

You should feel calm and soothed.

Expanding your lung care

Besides using your lungs according to their maker's instructions (as efficiently as possible) certain supplements can help to keep them in tip-top condition.

Fishing for omega-3

Omega-3 essential fatty acids (EFAs) are found in the flesh of oily fish – salmon, tuna, mackerel, sardines, and kippers are common sources. Essential to the heart and circulatory system, omega-3

EFAs also aid the lungs by helping to maintain healthy cell membranes within the alveoli.

Omega-3s also help to keep the blood running smoothly and freely, reducing risks of blood clots and (often fatal) *pulmonary embolism* – a fragment of clot or other debris released into the circulation which comes to rest in the lungs, blocking a major blood vessel.

In addition, clinical studies show that a preparation of omega-3 oils injected into a vein can dilute the thick, sticky mucus experienced by patients with cystic fibrosis and emphysema. Omega-3 oils have also proved useful to asthmatics, toning down their allergy symptoms and reducing lung inflammation.

Eat a 120–150 g portion of oily fish two or three times a week, or take three omega-3 capsules daily according to manufacturer's instructions during the revitalising stage of detox, and one or two (your choice) on a daily basis thereafter.

Getting the NAC (N-acetyl-cysteine)

Amino acids – the building blocks of proteins – include the sulphur-containing nutrient cysteine, which gives rise within the body to N-acetyl-cysteine (NAC). NAC is also obtained from protein foods in the diet, and not only does it positively feast upon free radicals, it also gives rise to glutathione – the most important cellular antioxidant known to man.

NAC is very useful to the lungs because it inhibits the development of cancer in tobacco smokers and counteracts the extra high yield of free radicals that can result from regular, vigorous exercise. It counteracts the flu virus, helps to maintain normal lung function and helps to protect the lungs from the effects of ageing and other damage. Take 500 mg daily during detox and on an everyday basis if you come into contact with a lot of cigarette smoke. You can obtain it from health food stores or pharmacists, but you may have to ask for it to be ordered for you.

Supporting Your Gut

The gut, which includes your intestines and bowels, is probably your most obvious waste disposal system. This powerful muscular pipe extends from the food pipe to the back passage, and handles all the myriad foods, drinks, and other junk we pile into it daily. It propels solids, liquids, and finally faeces along its length by waves of contraction, called *peristalsis.*

Going through the motions

The stomach is a roughly bean-shaped sac at rest but, being highly elastic, it assumes various shapes as it fills up with food and drink, of which it can hold up to two litres.

In a 24-hour period, the stomach's lining secretes about 3 litres of digestive fluid containing hydrochloric acid and enzymes – plus mucus to protect it from its own acid. The walls squeeze and mix the chewed and swallowed food with this powerful fluid, breaking it down to a pulp called chyme and splitting complex food molecules into smaller, simpler ones. After four to six hours, the stomach's contents are propelled in small, frequent squirts through the exit valve (pyloric sphincter) and into the duodenum, the first part of the small bowel. Here, chyme is mixed with alkaline secretions from the duodenal walls and the pancreas, and also with bile (a source of toxin elimination) which reaches it from the gall bladder and emulsifies fats.

The lining of the small bowel is covered with very small finger-like structures called villi that provide a huge absorption area for lique-fied food and drink. The villi are richly supplied with blood vessels, making it easy for nutrients and toxins to enter the bloodstream and travel to the liver (with a little of the emulsified fat entering the lymph system).

Waste matter, largely dietary fibre, gives the large bowel (colon) something solid on which to work. As the residue passes along towards the rectum, much of the remaining fluid is absorbed through the gut walls, and the residue forms firm stools. A percent-age of the fibre is broken down by friendly bacteria, while the rest soaks up gut toxins and prevents their re-absorption. Healthy bac-teria also counteract the unhealthy microbe colonies that produce intestinal toxins.

Giving your gut a helping hand

The basis of keeping your gut happy is to keep it active – that is: passing out waste regularly and effectively; limiting the amount of red meat you eat, because its breakdown products and toxins can cause gut disease and cancer; and keeping it well-nourished with suitable foods such as five-a-day portions of fresh fruit and vegeta-bles, and not too many hot spicy curries and other irritants. Your gut also needs to be kept well-hydrated, both for the sake of its own cells' health, and to render waste matter soft and easy to pass as motions.

Colonic irrigation – yes or no?

You have probably read of colonic irrigation in the press from time to time in connection with certain famous people.

In this practice or therapy (depending on your views), a tube is inserted into the back passage and water poured in, to sluice out the bowel and remove toxic waste. The theory is that most people's bowels are sluggish (due partly to a low fibre diet), and a toxic sludge is left, coating the colon's lining.

Some people swear by colonic irrigation; they're amazed at the quantity of foul debris that a single session can produce. However, huge colonies of friendly bacteria are also washed away in the process (truly chucking out the baby with the bath water). The so-called friendly bacteria encourage good overall gut function and keep the potentially harmful gut bacteria at bay. However, if you do decide to try colonic irrigation (and, let's face it, some people think it's the cat's whiskers), make sure that you go to a qualified, reputable therapist. Look under Naturopaths in Yellow Pages – colonic irrigation is a form of hydrotherapy (water therapy) which many naturopaths practise. Naturopaths use natural treatments such as sunlight, sea air, and water, to treat ailments.

Ingesting natural fibre and herbal supplements do such spring cleaning perfectly adequately – especially when followed by a rinsing-through with mineral water and probiotic supplements to rebalance the bacterial colonies.

Roughing it up with fibre

Fibre is the (generally) hard part of plants, which we nevertheless consume because of its benefits. Examples include bran (the husk and other fibrous part of wheat, oats, barley, rye, etc. – all grains), the structural parts of fruit and veg (such as the stalk and branches of broccoli, and similar veg), and the solid matter of pears, apples, and similar fruit. Practically without exception plant foods provide fibre, which is important to a healthy gut because it gives it something to grip. Water-soluble fibre is also of great importance because it buffers the lining of the gut against damage from sharp objects in food, and helps to absorb any toxins present in the gut. Pectin, the water-soluble fibre in many fruit (for example apples) is the best-known example.

Five plus portions of fresh fruit and vegetables each day provide adequate bulk for a healthy diet, but when detoxing, you need extra to ensure that the gut is swept as thoroughly as possible.

You can find a range of fibre-bulking agents in supermarkets and health food stores, and they come as seeds – for example, linseeds – as well as husks, granules, powders, and flakes. Follow the packet directions carefully (you usually take the supplement once or twice daily) and remember to drink extra water while using them because they absorb sufficient water to cause a shortage in the bowel, if you drink too little.

Psyllium husks (*Plantago psyllium*, guar gum) are an excellent choice for absorbing bowel toxins. They swell up to 15 times their bulk when mixed with water so they also have a natural laxative effect. Also, as dietary fibre provides nutrients for gut bacteria, the useful bugs multiply more efficiently, too. Remember to vary your choice of fibre from time to time as the bacteria get used to one type and begin to break it down so effectively that some of the benefits of taking it may be lost.

Encouraging bacteria

Probiotics are the natural gut-friendly bacteria you need to colonise and balance your bowel. Prebiotics such as garlic, onions, wheat, barley, bananas, honey, and tomatoes have in common a substance called *fructo-oligosaccarides (FOs)* – a carbohydrate which cannot be digested or absorbed by humans but which promotes its colonisation of the bowel by healthy, useful bugs.

Healthy quantities of beneficial gut bacteria help to remove toxins from the large bowel, to balance digestive processes, and to reduce the risks of infection with harmful gut bacteria such as *Salmonella* and *E. coli.*

Live bio-yoghurt is the commonest source of this type of bacteria, but commercial yoghurts containing *Lactobacillus acidophilus* and similar species vary in the number of live bacteria they actually provide. Excellent sources include homemade yoghurt produced with freeze-dried acidophilus, fermented milk drinks with lactobacilli, and supplements that guarantee a specified number of bacteria per dose.

During a detox regimen, you are better off taking a supplement whose useful bacteria quota is more reliable than that of yoghurt. Choose one that supplies 10 million to 2 billion colony-forming units per dose. A good option is to take such a supplement for at least a month according to manufacturer's instructions and repeat several times a year when you feel the need.

Flushing, then soothing with aloe vera

How much extra water should you drink when detoxing? Calculating the quantity is difficult but, assuming you are using a fibre supplement as advised in the preceding 'Roughing it up with fibre' section, you can try an extra litre each day and see how you go.

Novice detoxers sometimes object to drinking this much water on the grounds that they will always be visiting the loo. Well . . . no. The point is that the fibre actually absorbs a sizeable percentage of your fluid intake, leaving you with softer, bulkier stools but not necessarily much of an increased urine output.

Aloe vera juice is made from the gel of the *Aloe barbardensis* – a cactus-type plant native to Africa, used in herbal medicine for at least 2,000 years. The gel contains a unique array of vitamins and minerals, amino acids, and enzymes in addition to soapy saponin compounds that help disperse fatty deposits, and lignin fibres that absorb toxins and fluids from the gut and add bulk to the stools. Aloe vera is best known for its soothing properties (many people use it to treat burns) and a great aid to the gut during detox, when the gut lining may protest (that is, get slightly inflamed or sore) due to the brand new eating regimen and the increased load of toxins it is being required to expel.

Aloe vera is good for detoxing because the antioxidant vitamins and minerals strengthen the bowel lining when your body is dealing with an excess of toxins during a detox. The water-soluble fibre (lignins) add natural bulk to encourage the bowel to work briskly; and the saponin natural soaps start the cleansing process of the bowel lining when the excess waste matter has been evacuated.

Avoid Aloe vera if you are pregnant or breast-feeding because it triggers uterine contractions.

Part II
Detoxing Your Diet

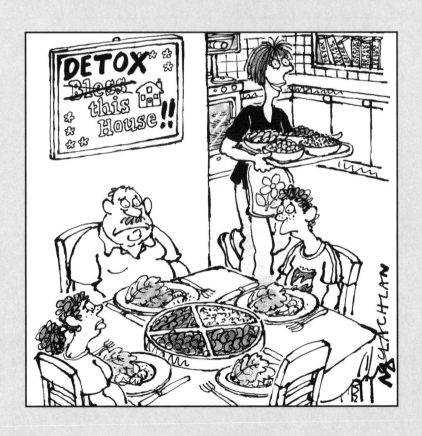

In this part . . .

You are what you eat is true. Food can give you healthy benefits and cause toxins to enter your body, so it pays to take care with what you eat. In Chapter 4 I guide you through the principles of healthy (and enjoyable) eating, and show you the common mistakes that can lead to you eating far less healthily than you imagine.

In Chapter 5 I give you details of useful, healthy foods to eat during detox, which are also of benefit to your health generally. In Chapter 6 I tell you about the foods that you must avoid during when detoxing, including how and why it's necessary to give them a miss.

Chapter 4

Detoxing Essentials

*D*etox – short for *detoxification* – gets rid of the impurities or toxins that, over time, accumulate in your body from a number of sources including the environment (such as in the water supply, the atmosphere and foods weighed down with chemical colourings, flavourings and other additives). Detox relies mainly on dietary measures, replacing foods and drinks loaded with fat, refined sugar, caffeine, and other substances with alternatives that promote and support the cleansing process.

If you do nothing else, switching to a predominantly organic diet and eating foods that are raw or only lightly cooked will get your detox off to a great start.

Detox Now!

Detox is currently trendy. You may have read about it in connection with the streamlined, glossy appearances of fashion and pop icons such as Sadie Frost, Juliette Binoche, and Patsy Kensit. Detox is the method new mums Victoria Beckham, Julia Roberts, Gwyneth Paltrow, and Anna Friel used to shed their surplus pounds speedily. Yet detox is not new – fasting is mentioned in the Bible as a source of purification, and numerous saints and gurus followed liquids-only regimens to heighten their experience of ecstasy.

Don't worry, though – you don't need to be a saint, pop star, or model mum to benefit from an internal cleansing. And there is absolutely no need to fast – in fact, a liquids-only diet, whether of water or fruit and vegetable juices, can be a severe shock to the system and make you feel exhausted and weak.

Cleansing your body of toxins using a detox helps to boost energy levels, improve your memory, alertness and concentration, clear your complexion, and strengthen and condition your hair. Vague but persistent symptoms such as a stuffy nose, bags below the eyes, premature wrinkles, headaches, drowsiness, aching muscles, and constipation also tend to disappear with its use.

The three stages of detoxing are cleansing, balancing, and fortifying.

Cleansing

Detoxing cleanses by encouraging your body to eliminate toxins swiftly and efficiently. You can read about the cleansing process in more detail, including the need to drink eight to ten glasses of water daily, in Chapter 3, Supporting Your Detox Organs.

Foods and drinks of this stage of detox provide a gentle start to your detox programme. Suitable foods, and others to avoid, are discussed in Chapters 5 and 6 respectively, and you can read about organic foods further on in this chapter.

Balancing

Detox helps to balance your body nutritionally after the cleansing stage has become established. This means providing you with all the essential nutrients you need in the same sort of foods but supplemented by dietary nutrients. Literally dozens of essential nutrients and other supplements exist that you can take for their balancing effect; and are detailed in Chapter 11.

Fortifying

Having offloaded a lot of toxins and increased your inner harmony, you probably want to enhance these newfound benefits in as many ways as you can. Essentially this means banishing toxic habits such as smoking and over-drinking, and instead eating cleansing, balancing organic foods with their wide spectrum of vitamins, minerals, and unique phytochemicals – plant constituents such as the chlorophyll in algae and bright green plants.

For optimal effects, you should also minimise negative stress in your lifestyle and environment. In Chapters 8 and 9, I show you how to check yourself for stress symptoms and how to cope with sources of stress whenever you encounter them.

Negative stress (the sort that exhausts you with fatigue and tension rather than buoying you up with goals and challenges) actually increases the numbers of free radicals in your tissues and exacerbates the damage they can produce. Besides relaxation and improved sleep, you could try a number of supplements, which counterbalance stress's harmful effects and improve your ability to deal with stress successfully. You can read about the supplements in Chapter 11.

Do you need to detox?

Beauty is more than skin deep. Whatever your figure and facial contours, you *can* have healthily shining hair; blemish-free skin; clear, sparkling eyes; and be bursting with energy and vitality.

But do we ever achieve this? As the pace of modern life gets ever faster and demands on us grow, everyone tends to eat too much fat, sugar, and low-fibre convenience food packed with artificial additives. Some of us smoke, many people find it hard to relax, we nearly all suffer from the effects of stress, and every single one of us is exposed to environmental pollutants.

You may perhaps add to this list a high alcohol intake, lots of high-caffeine coffee, fizzy drinks, chronic dehydration, lack of fresh air and exercise, and poor-quality sleep. Is it any wonder that for much of the time, you look and feel terribly below par – or perhaps just terrible?

Chronic toxin overload causes premature ageing, and increases the risks of an untimely death from heart disease, stroke, diabetes, obesity, or cancer. But life on the run is an inescapable part of living today for most people. Can you alter this? If so, how?

The first step in your detox program is acknowledging that you put your body under enormous strain. Perhaps you're used to feeling tired and below par, so notice nothing amiss. But, unaided, your body can only go so far. An annual or bi-annual detox can help to reduce the risks of all the diseases listed above.

Your body strives, 24/7, to eliminate toxins with a variety of Herculean efforts:

✔ Your liver and kidneys neutralise and excrete toxic overloads via bile and in urine, respectively.

✔ Your colon (large bowel) struggles to eliminate low-fibre, toxin-ridden waste.

✔ Your skin perspires, excretes oil, and sheds dead cells to throw off debris.

✔ Your lymphatic system, small vessels and lymph nodes situated throughout the body, filters off toxic waste and dead cells from your blood, tissues and organs.

What happens when these stalwarts fail? As toxins accumulate, you can develop a number of possible symptoms. You may, for example, become exhausted, lack your usual stamina, catch colds and other infections more easily, have a dull complexion, plus sundry aches and pains.

If a toxic overload develops unhindered, you run an increased risk of more serious complaints such as clogged arteries, bowel disorders, gallstones, a dysfunctional liver, obesity, diabetes, and cancer.

Detoxing cleanses your body by encouraging it to eliminate toxins swiftly and efficiently. Chapter 3 talks more about the cleansing process, including the need to drink eight to ten glasses of water daily.

Everything you eat and drink during a detox programme is specifically chosen to enhance the three phases of cleanse, balance, and strengthen. The fewer foods you eat, the easier it is to ensure optimal results, and the less likely you are to be tempted to stray from the programme.

Substance abusers and detox

Detoxing is also central to the treatment of alcoholics and other substance abusers who suffer withdrawal symptoms as toxins clear from the system.

The detox plan written up for hospitalised patients includes major tranquillisers to ease pain, sweating, raving, and other suffering. Replacing one set of toxins with another, you may think! But the sedatives are tailed off as soon as the person is ready, and restorative nutrients of protein, vitamins, and minerals are prescribed from the start of the care plan.

There's a saying that there is no gain without pain and that's one way of looking at detoxing, but I am not sure that it's the most alluring. You may find, as do many people, that you have to 'psyche yourself up' in order to commit to a detox plan in whose outcome you have to have faith because it cannot be measured objectively.

Saying that you mean to detox, is one thing, but the prospect of kicking your coffee habit, forgoing fats, signing off from sugar and trouncing your takeaways can prove terribly daunting. It's just too easy to postpone actually *starting* detox to an endless succession of tomorrows. This book, however, is emphatically about doing – not procrastinating about – detox, which is why I like to focus on how much better you'll feel without your toxin-laden favourites, rather than on how deprived you may feel without them.

Going Organic

Many of the advantages of organic produce and other food types you may not have thought about, such as raw, wild, and others selected for their colours.

Organic fruit and veg contain on average twice the vitamins, trace elements, essential fatty acids, and phytochemicals (plant nutrients) of non-organic produce. They are also free from chemicals, such as herbicides, pesticides, and so on, making them purer, and therefore better for you.

Equally, they tend to taste a great deal better. Organic foods are generally fresher than non-organically grown produce because they are allowed to ripen naturally in the soil or on the stem. Non-organic vegetables and fruit are often plucked long before they're ripe, and stored at low temperatures for months while awaiting transport – often to the other side of the Earth.

 You can avoid paying a prohibitive price – and find great foods – by buying locally from markets, farm shops and allotment owners. Check whether the growers spray their crops and, if so, with what (see Chapter 2 for advice on what to avoid).

Another excellent source of organic fruit and veg are keen garden-ers, often living within a stone's throw of large cities. Many organic farmers now advertise on the Internet, and you can have fresh garden and farm produce delivered practically anywhere in the UK at 24 hours' notice. Check out www.organicfood.co.uk/shopping/index.html to start your search.

Going Raw

Raw foods, that is, raw fruit and veg, nuts and seeds, have much to offer you when detoxing; and also when maintaining the benefits of detox thereafter.

The benefits

The benefits stem mainly from the effect upon the body of essential nutrients in their natural forms.

Living nutrients

Vital nutrients, plant enzymes and other natural plant constituents enter your body in their original form. Vitamins and minerals are able to exert their full antioxidant effect, energising your immune system during detox, and helping to protect it against free radicals.

Free radicals are super-charged oxygen fragments generated in the body's tissues in excessive numbers by the presence of toxins (which become extra-active during detox, because detox 'rounds them up' and prepares them for elimination by your excretory organs).

Free radicals damage cells throughout the body, contributing to early ageing signs such as wrinkly skin, and degenerative diseases such as arthritis, heart disease and cancer.

Forceful fibre

Fibre's full effect is obtained – and felt – when you eat raw foods. Some fibre is inactivated, that is, made less effective, by cooking, but raw fruit and vegetables supply plant fibre in its natural state. It can then act on the bowel, absorbing released toxins harmlessly into the faeces (stools), and swelling with water to trigger effective evacuation.

Studies show that Africans in undeveloped communities suffer far less than people in the West, from bowel disorders such as diverticulitis, irritable bowel syndrome, chronic constipation, and cancer of the colon. The researchers conclude that the Africans' relatively high intake of raw foods and natural fibre is largely responsible.

Regular and effective bowel elimination is a focal point of successful detox.

Energy boost

Food energy levels are much higher in raw foods than in their cooked or processed counterparts. This refers to the life force present in living plant foods, and recognised particularly by holistic practitioners.

Kirlian photography captures pictures on film of the electromagnetic field around living plant (and other) cells, now believed by many orthodox scientists to represent their vitality and energy levels.

Both Kirlian photography and similar methods of detection, show far stronger, more balanced and more life-enhancing force fields around fresh, uncooked fruit and veg, than the fields surrounding the same foods when cooked or processed.

Hundreds of thousands of anecdotal accounts attest to the energy-giving effects of eating raw food; in fact, the original muesli was designed by the Swiss doctor, Bircher-Benner, to help heal his patients of life-threatening diseases.

Weight loss

Raw fruit and vegetables are a great weight loss aid. This is partly due to their enhanced nutritional benefits, and partly to chewing and digesting plant food in its raw state. It fills you up more quickly, and helps to combat cravings for sugar, fat and addictive artificial food additives such as the flavour-enhancer monosodium glutamate.

Many seasoned detoxers eat a large raw salad every day, both during and between detoxing. A plate of raw salad foods or lightly cooked vegetables certainly reduces your appetite for subsequent courses.

Going Wild

It depends what you mean by wild! I certainly wouldn't suggest turning to the countryside and picking handfuls of unappetising-looking weeds and other greenery – even if you are certain that you have identified it correctly.

However, a number of wild foods are easy to find and their inclusion in your detox programme adds interest, variety and nutritional value. Here are a few for you to consider:

Bilberries

Bilberries (known as blueberries in the USA), are found in Britain in woodland scrub, and are chock-full of anthrocyanins – powerful antioxidants that pep up the immune defence system and benefit small blood vessels, especially those supplying the retina at the back of the eye.

Fungi

Unless you are a fungi specialist, don't eat any fungi until they have been positively identified. Mistakes cost lives. This said, many interesting mushrooms and puffballs can be found in woodlands and similar areas. They supply a range of vitamins and minerals (depending on their type), mainly protein, B complex and K vitamins, copper and other minerals, plus fibre for easy bowel movements. Their textures and flavours add interest to a range of savoury dishes and soups.

Blackberries

Many people look forward to the autumn, for the chance to pick and enjoy wild blackberries. This fruit contains antioxidant anthrocyanins, as well as vitamin C and other nutrients.

Blackberries also improve the flavour of such foods as porridge, muesli, fruit salads, and cooked rice dishes. They make a wholesome, non-fattening snack between detox meals, and can be incorporated into smoothies, milk shakes, and other fruit recipes to great effect.

You can find blackberries in most British hedgerows from August/September onwards. They are fun to pick (so much nutritional value for free!), and need little attention other than washing and picking over. Just try to choose blackberries growing in field or hedgerow as far as possible from car and other transport pollution.

Crabapples

This delightful little fruit is both beautiful, and chock-full of detox nutrients. Crabapples are a kind of wild apple, occasionally cultivated but more often found 'in the wild' in country hedgerows, and woodland.

Slightly larger than, and coloured like the celebrated 'white' variety of cultivated cherry, crabapples appear from mid-summer to mid-autumn. Their pale yellow or cream skin has an evocative, rosy blush, and they can be picked as firm, glossy fruit like plums and greengages.

Crabapples supply vitamins A and C, calcium, iron, and a little fibre. Being sugar- (and fat-) free, they can be lightly stewed with other sweet fruit, or just used to adorn your detox dishes when entertaining.

Going For Colour

The more interesting and attractive food looks, the more appetising; but choosing a range of coloured foods when detoxing is important in other ways.

Rainbow effect

Think of a rainbow when selecting salad foods. Bright green and red salad leaves add moisture, vitamins, and vitamin C. Purple beetroot supplies fibre, beta carotenes (the coloured pigment), and a range of minerals including potassium, calcium, magnesium, and iron.

Beetroot are also said to calm the nerves (possibly due to their calcium and magnesium content) and to help build new red blood cells. You can also eat their leaves, raw or lightly steamed, in a salad or other dish.

Fresh sweet corn kernels provide a cheerful splash of yellow, plus fibre, starch and natural sugar. Grated raw carrot contributes its orange hue, and is rich in beta carotene (pro-vitamin A). Grated red cabbage supplies a blue colour (uncommon in plant foods) if you lightly steam it first.

Cabbages give you a range of vitamins including vitamin C, potassium and other minerals, fibre, and the nutrient once called vitamin U, because of its soothing effect upon an irritated, inflamed stomach lining and peptic ulcers.

You can also scatter your salad or other dishes with seeds. Greyish-green pumpkin seeds supply a satisfying, nutty flavour and energy, plus omega-6 oils and a little protein, and are extremely rich in the minerals manganese, magnesium, iron, copper, zinc, and phosphorus, as well as tryptophan – the amino acid (protein building block) needed by the brain to manufacture serotonin which helps to combat depression, insomnia, and anxiety disorders.

Colourful cooked foods

You can apply the same rainbow principle to stir-fries, grills, braised dishes, and barbecues – think of purple aubergines (which turn a dark purple rather than black when cooked), and crimson tomatoes (which you can cook, for instance for breakfast on whole-grain toast) or serve sliced as a salad, alongside a cooked dish.

Tomatoes are richer than any other plant foods in lycopene, a phytonutrient or plant constituent proven in clinical trials studies to help to combat cancer of the prostate, bladder, and other organs.

Spinach, rich in iron and magnesium, is worth trying again if you disliked it as a child and haven't eaten it since. It goes slightly darker when cooked, and is most delicious when lightly cooked and carefully pressed in a sieve to remove all surplus water.

Many cooked dishes tend to be darker than their raw counterparts, and you can add contrast with creamy white chopped or grated almonds, macadamias, cashews, brazils or other nuts, and lightly cooked sunshine kernels or fresh sweet corn.

Nuts are relatively high in calories because they have a high oil content, but this consists mostly of the healthy monounsaturated type like that found in olive oil. Nuts are low-GI (so provide energy without bumping up your blood sugar all of a sudden), and they also supply protein and fibre.

Going Probiotic

Probiotics are natural gut-friendly bacteria that you need to colonise and balance your bowel. Excellent sources include homemade yoghurt made with freeze-dried acidophilus, fermented milk drinks with lactobacilli, and supplements that guarantee a specified number of bacteria per capsule, tablet or measure of powder. Choose one that supplies from between 10 million to 2 billion colony-forming units per dose. A good option is to take such a supplement, according to the manufacturer's instructions, for at least a month and repeat several times a year when you feel the need.

Healthy quantities of beneficial gut bacteria help to remove toxins from the large bowel, balance digestive processes, and reduce the risks of infection from harmful gut bacteria such as *Salmonella* and *E. coli*. Live bio-yoghurt is the most common source but commercial yoghurts containing *Lactobacillus acidophilus* and similar species vary in the number of live bacteria they actually provide. During a detox regimen, you are better off taking a supplement whose useful bacteria quota is more reliable.

Growing Your Own

You may already belong to the swelling numbers of people who grow much of their own produce. Yes, it *is* easier to dial your local supermarket and have them deliver a box of greens, but DIY veg and fruit are infinitely more fun, amazingly healthy, and a good deal cheaper.

If you have never gardened before, whet your appetite by watching one of the many excellent gardening programmes on TV, or buy a book about it (you can often find 'offers' on large, popular, well-known titles once they've been released for a few months. Look in the catalogues of postal book clubs, on-line, and in local bookshops, as well as the stationery department of large supermarkets).

Garden centres want to sell their wares and, for this reason alone, are generally happy to give advice about organic gardening aids, suitable plants, and the sort of tools to buy. And you are almost bound to have gardening friends or family members who would gladly help you get started on this fascinating and health-boosting hobby.

Allotments

Allotments have never been more popular. Waiting lists of up to two years are common in many places, especially in large cities. But imagine you've reached the top of the list and regularly bring home delicious fresh radishes and beetroot, cabbages and salad leaves, tomatoes and broccoli – not to mention most gardeners' pride and joy, new potatoes?

Allotments have other benefits besides fresh garden produce. They can be great meeting places for people with similar interests, and the 'little hut' that many owners have on site to keep their tools in, also provides a legitimate hideout when you want to escape from home for a few hours (what could be more praiseworthy than toiling under a hot sun – or in wind and rain – for the good of your family?)

Meanwhile, as watching (even organic) vegetables and fruit grow is not much more inspiring than watching paint dry, you can be sitting in your deckchair out of the weather, refreshing yourself with a cup of tea (think vacuum flask or Primus stove), or tasting a sweet tomato or handful of strawberries or raspberries picked seconds before.

You can also entertain fellow allotment owners in your hut, picking up tips and exchanging gardening (and other) news. Most old-timers are happy to help novice gardeners, because everyone likes an excuse to hold forth upon their pet subject.

Gardens and patios

Of course there's no need for an allotment if you have a garden large enough for vegetable beds, embellished, perhaps, with a cucumber frame or small greenhouse. Even if you haven't (and doubt that you'd have time to grow anything in it if you had), pots on a patio or a window box require little looking-after, compared with the trophies they produce for the picking. They also require less watering than a full garden.

Is there room just outside your back door for a growbag for nice crops of juicy tomatoes? Or maybe you'd prefer a specially designed grow-pot, available from garden centres, supermarkets and other outlets, in which you can cultivate almost any plant food nowadays, from sweet peppers to baby aubergines, courgettes to strawberries, blueberries to olives.

Not forgetting the kitchen sink . . . !

Well, not the sink exactly, but the window sill above it, on which you can place a row of flower pots growing salad leaves, fresh herbs, cress, and small tomato plants. And you needn't move an inch to water them, or wash your hands afterwards!

Chapter 5

What To Eat – and Why

*K*nowing what to eat and, just as essentially, why, is vital for a successful detox. How can you follow a stringent plan for cleansing your body of toxins and replacing them with beneficial nutrients if you're unaware of the benefits of particular foods and the hazards of others?

In this chapter, I look at carbohydrates and the importance of choosing the low G.I. (glycaemic index) variety. I also consider dietary fats – to help you distinguish between the safe and the unsafe – and proteins which, although occasionally over-stressed by trendy weight-loss diets, are vital to life, health, vitality, and well-being.

Energising with Carbohydrates

Carbohydrates are the body's chief source of energy. They give the body glucose – either directly because they contain it, or indirectly through their starch content – which is converted into glucose by enzymes in the mouth and the small bowel. Glucose is absolutely essential to brain and other vital organ function; human life is unsustainable for more than a few minutes without glucose.

Glucose, a fundamental body food, is burned in the cells of the body to release energy, carbon dioxide, and, as a by-product, a little water.

Finding the right source of carbohydrates

Nutritional experts place a great deal of importance on wholefood carbohydrates – the kind you eat when detoxing (and, hopefully, at other times, too!) Wholefood carbs are valuable because they contain all the food's original nutrients – with 'nothing added and nothing taken away'. An example is wholewheat flour made from the entire grain, therefore giving you both wheat germ and the full fibre content. Another is brown rice. Both these differ from their white counterparts, which provide far fewer nutrients and little, if any, fibre.

Good sources of wholefood carbohydrates are oats, rye, barley, as well as wheat, and products made from them. Pulses are also excellent choices, chickpeas, for example, along with lentils, peas and beans, and other sources such as sweet potatoes, fresh sweet corn, nuts and seeds.

All these are yummy foods in their own right (besides supplying you with many nutrients), but you also have to ensure that you are taking in enough of them daily to meet your body's needs.

Getting the right amount of carbohydrate

Nowadays, nutritionists generally agree that carbohydrates need to supply 50– 60 per cent of your daily caloric intake. So, if you are taking in 2,000 calories daily, then 1,000–1,100 of those calories need to come from the natural starches and sugars that carbohydrates provide. I give the example of 2,000 calories because this is approximately the amount of energy adults need to derive daily from their diet. Men need slightly more than women, say, 2,250–2,500 calories, or even more if they do heavy physical work. Women need between 1,800–2,400 calories daily, also depending upon the amount of energy they use. Personal body structure, age, and metabolic rate (rate of burning food fuel) also come into the picture. A 10-stone labourer would need fewer calories than a 15-stone labourer doing the same work, while a 90-year-old woman would need fewer calories than her 20-year-old great-granddaughter.

Assuming that your daily intake of carbohydrates amounts to 1,000 calories (for the sake of simple calculation), and knowing that carbohydrates supply 4 calories per gram, you need to eat around 250 grams of carbohydrates every day.

The wholefood grains and cereals discussed above provide your main sources of healthy carbohydrates. When not detoxing, you almost certainly include small amounts of refined carbohydrates such as sweets, chocolate, and honey in your everyday eating. But where carbs are introduced on your detox plan, you obtain them from the wholegrain sources.

Why are detoxers, and healthy eaters generally, so wary of refined (white) sugar and food containing it? Well, it isn't just a change of 'naughty but nice' into 'naughty and therefore a no-no' by doom-laden nutritionists bent on spoiling your fun. A little refined sugar, outside of detox, is unlikely to harm you, although don't eat it when you are detoxing. This is because sugar-laden processed and junk foods can make you feel ill, and affect your body's ability to deal with fats and carbohydrates generally. Have you, for instance, heard of the glucose high? If not, read the next section of this book.

The glucose high

Being 'high' on glucose is partly responsible for the renowned feel-good effect of chocolate, and can lift your spirits when low. It can also be useful in the short term if you have to race for a bus or train, or have a challenging situation to face, when you need immediate access to instant energy. In the long run though, a high of glucose does you no good.

Your blood glucose level falls as rapidly as it rises when you eat refined (that is, non-wholefood) carbs, because after the glucose has swooshed into your system, insulin (a hormone produced by the pancreas gland close to your stomach) chases it out of your bloodstream and into your cells.Your blood glucose level plummets suddenly as a result, and this can make you sweat profusely, feel shaky and faint, and find your heart racing at nineteen to the dozen. These unpleasant symptoms caused by low blood glucose (hypoglycaemia) can force you to sit down wherever you happen to be, or urgently seek fresh air. The experience can be scary if you do not know its cause.

As your glucose level drops, you'll also lose your high, euphoric mood, and probably crave another quick 'glucose hit'.

An important way that detox foods help balance the body is by guarding against blood glucose highs and lows. The majority of the unrefined carbohydrates you eat during detox (such as brown rice, wholegrain breads and cereals, jacket potatoes, and wholewheat pasta) have a low G.I. – glycaemic index – rating. This low rating indicates that these foods release their sugar and starches slowly into your bloodstream, thus keeping your blood glucose (sugar) level on an even keel.

High fibre, low G.I. foods raise your blood glucose g-r-a-d-u-a-l-l-y, providing a more sustained source of energy and avoiding the unhealthy highs and lows – they are real balancing foods! Low G.I. foods also require far less insulin than high G.I. foods to deal with the sugars they release. Abnormally raised levels of insulin are therefore avoided. Excess levels of this hormone, over time, are known to promote obesity and increase the risks of heart disease, cancer, and other fatal illnesses.

An important way that detox foods help to balance the body is by guarding against blood glucose highs and lows. The majority of the unrefined carbohydrates you eat during detox (such as brown rice, wholegrain breads and cereals, jacket potatoes, and wholewheat pasta) have a low G.I. – glycaemic index – rating. This low rating indicates that these foods release their sugar and starches slowly into your bloodstream, thus keeping your blood glucose (sugar) level on an even keel.

On the other hand, foods with a high G.I. rating (such as refined sugar, white bread, and white/refined grain products) contain little or no fibre and consequently release their sugars and starches soon after digestion starts. High G.I. foods bump up your blood glucose level. This may be useful shortly before a sprint when you need an immediate fund of ready energy, but it does you little good in the normal run of things!

When detoxing, choose foods with a low to medium G.I. And as a general health rule, if you're eating foods with a high G.I. rating, combine them with low G.I. ones in the same meal.

Table 5-1 is a guide to the G.I. value of familiar foods.

Table 5-1	Glycaemic Index of Select Foods
Food	*G.I. Rating*
Apples	38
Apricots	57
French baguette	95
Organic baked beans	42
Bananas	52

Food	G.I. Rating
Barley	25
Butter beans	36
Haricot beans	38
Kidney beans	29
Soy beans	15
White bread	70
Wholegrain rye bread	42
Wholegrain wheat bread	77
Carrots	47
Chick peas	42
Cornflakes	81
Grapefruit	25
Grapes	46
Honey	55
Lentils	29
Skimmed milk	32
Whole milk	27
Oats	58
Oranges	42
Parsnips	97
White pasta	40
Wholemeal pasta	37
Peaches	42
Peanuts	14
Peas	51
Popcorn (low fat)	53
Baked potatoes	85
Sweet potatoes	54

(continued)

Table 5-1 *(continued)*

Food	G.I. Rating
Raisins	64
Brown rice	55
White rice	74
Sweetcorn	55
Weetabix	68

You may not fancy brown rice (for example) when you've always been used to the white variety. But brown rice's low G.I. and nutrient value does make it the superior food. You can also expect to enjoy its nutty flavour, texture, and fill-you-up factor; it does take longer to cook than refined (white) rice (25–30 minutes as opposed to 10–12 minutes), but this is true of most low-G.I. natural foods as opposed to their high-G.I. and/or processed counterparts.

You can get other new food experiences from low G.I. eating. As you can see from Table 5-1, a French baguette has a G.I. of 95, while wholegrain rye bread's G.I. of 42 is almost half this value. Look for Westphalian rye bread, also sold as Pumpernickel, in all large supermarkets. It has a rich, brown smell a bit like pipe tobacco, it's deliciously moist and crustless, and its strong flavour is complemented by many natural foods such as mashed avocado or reduced fat hummus or goat's cheese.

Greasing the Wheels with Fats and Oils

You've no doubt heard and read that fats are bad news. Fattening foods lead to obesity, a serious disorder affecting millions of people in all developed countries. Sufferers run a greatly increased risk of high blood pressure and other circulatory disorders. In fact, fat not only promotes obesity (with its built-in, high mortality risk), it also sidles into your arteries, whether you're fat or not, clogging them up and triggering coronary heart attacks and strokes. Clearly, the less you have to do with fat, the better, you may think!

As usual, where you body is concerned, things aren't quite as simple as they seem. A certain amount of fat is essential in maintaining healthy tissues, nerves, and brain cells, and in manufacturing hormones and other vital compounds. A totally fat-free diet (were such a thing possible) would be disastrous because your body would lack essential fatty acids (EFAs), which strengthen and preserve all cell membranes and are used to make prostaglandins – short-lived, hormone-like cellular chemicals. Prostaglandin deficiency has been linked to numerous disorders including ADHD (attention deficit hyperactivity disorder), eczema, arthritis, premenstrual tension, and menopausal symptoms.

Getting the right amount – and the right type – of fat

The carbohydrates and protein in your food supply just 4 calories per gram while fats provide 9 calories per gram making fats twice as fattening as these other food groups.

When determining how much fat you need, it all comes back to balance! Nutritionists advise that the total amount of fat you consume daily should not exceed more than 30 per cent of your daily calorie intake. So, if you consume 2,000 calories, not more than 660 should come from fats and oils. Bearing in mind that fat supplies 9 calories per gram, then your total daily fat intake needs to average around 73 grams.

Seventy-three grams may sound generous when you consider the size of a piece of butter weighing this amount, and how far you can make it stretch! But hidden fats abound in nearly all processed foods and junk snacks, and it's easy to reach and exceed your advised daily quota without eating any 'visible' fats such as butter, margarine, cream, or fried food.

Finding the right source for fats

When detoxing, you need to avoid unhealthy fats and oils and choose healthy ones.

Unhealthy fats

The first type of unhealthy fat is the saturated type found in full-fat dairy foods, and in and around red meat. It tends to form fatty plaques (patches) on the walls of arteries, clogging their channels and interfering with the blood's circulation. These fatty patches also 'invite' the formation of clots, especially when the blood flow through them is reduced to a relative trickle. *Some* saturated fat occurs in nearly all plant oils but the quantity is generally negligible. As a result, vital organs like the heart and brain run short of nutrients and oxygen (carried by blood); large clots can impede the blood flow totally. Narrowed arteries supplying the heart (for example) cause angina or chest pain, and a clot within them causes a heart attack.

The second form of unhealthy fat is the trans variety and hydrogenated oils, into which healthy plant oils are changed when heated in cooking, or processed to a high temperature. You find these in margarine (for example), and many processed foods which claim correctly that they are made from plant oil as opposed to saturated fat, but do not let on that high temperatures have changed the original healthy polyunsaturates into the harmful sort.

Trans fats and hydrogenated oils are harmful because they have an anti-vitamin effect, combating the healthy effects of antioxidants and attacking the immune defence system (thereby leading to degenerative disorders like early ageing, cancer, arthritis, and other complaints).

Healthy fats

You find healthy fats in the oils of plants, fish, seeds, and nuts. Two kinds that you will have heard of are monounsaturated and polyunsaturated.

Olive oil contains a monounsaturated oil named oleic acid. Monounsaturated oils differ in chemical structure to polyunsaturated plant oils, (for example, safflower, sunflower), but nevertheless provide similar benefits. These include reducing the cholesterol in the blood and promoting a healthy heart and arteries, thereby reducing the risks of a heart attack or stroke. Monounsaturated oils also provide potassium, calcium, and antioxidants vitamin E and polyphenols.

Cold-pressed plant oils are rich in omega-6 essential fatty acids. These are the polyunsaturated variety that are beneficial to the immune system and have a huge range of vital actions throughout the body's tissues and organs. The cold-pressing process leaves healthy essential fatty acids (EFAs) intact whereas commercial refining strips out the EFAs. Cold-pressed oils retain most of their healthy properties when used for cooking, if you subject them to as low a temperature and for as short a time as you can manage for whatever you are preparing. This is one reason why stir-frying (which takes a few minutes only) is a healthy cooking option.

Good sources of cold-pressed plant oils include safflower, linseed, sunflower, and corn oil, all of which are rich in omega-6 essential fatty acids, especially alpha-linoleic acid, which aids prostaglandin production (this helps to balance the hormone levels and keep heart, circulation, skin, and other organs healthy).

Further 'healthy oil' choices include nuts and seeds, although the quantity you are likely to obtain from these sources is relatively low.

Walnuts and their oil have a 7 to 1 ratio of polyunsaturated to saturated fats (all plant oils contain a small quantity of saturated fat). They also provide cholesterol-reducing plant factors and omega-6 EFAs and have the highest antioxidant action of all nuts, followed by almonds and pistachios. Eating a handful of walnuts (or a salad dressing made using walnut oil) four or five times a week can significantly lower blood cholesterol levels and reduce your risks of suffering a heart attack by between 15 and 51 per cent.

Catching fish oils

Beneficial fat and oil sources include oily fish rich in omega-3 essential fatty acids (EFAs), especially two called Eicosapentaenoic acid (EPA) and Docosahexaenoic acid (DHA), which are necessary to the brain and central nervous system. The British Nutritional Foundation (BNF) suggests eating at least 300 grams of oily fish every week.

Good oily fish choices include mackerel, herrings, tuna, salmon, kippers, and sardines.

 Make sure that you buy organic fish from sea or freshwater sources declared organic by the Soil Association. Alternatively, if you dislike fish but are not allergic to it, you can take a fish oil supplement from a mainstream company, following the label directions as to the dose.

Cracking seeds, nuts, and veg sources

Other useful oils come from nuts and seeds, an excellent example being pumpkin seeds.

 Pumpkin seeds and pumpkin oil are rich sources of omega-6 and omega-3 EFAs. You can purchase the oil online from various Internet sites. Pumpkin seeds, eaten as a snack or added to muesli, salads, soups, or other dishes, are an excellent way to obtain a healthy source of essential fatty acids.

Building Up Proteins

Protein is found in meat, eggs, and beans and is broken down during digestion into its component amino acids – the building blocks from which new tissues and cells are formed. Amino acids also contribute to the manufacture of enzymes, hormones, and other metabolic substances.

This rebuilding process is especially important during detox because as the old tissue and cells are removed, your body urgently requires replacement materials.

Getting the right amount of protein

Nutritional guidelines advise that proteins supply 10–20 per cent of daily calorie intake. If you take in 2,000 calories daily, then 200–400 calories need to come from protein. Like carbohydrates, protein supplies 4 calories per gram, so you're looking at eating 50–100 grams of protein.

First-class protein sources such as red meat, game, fowl, fish, eggs, and dairy products supply the majority of the amino acids that human beings require, including the eight essential ones that we cannot synthesise for ourselves from other sources.

Second-class proteins provide some, although not all, of the essential amino acids, and include wholegrain rice, other vegetables, soya products, pulses, beans, and nuts. You can obtain the full range of essential amino acids you need by eating foods from the main vegetarian groups: pulses, grains, cereals, nuts and seeds.

Detox programmes tend to cut down on red meat, eggs, and dairy products, so you need to ensure that you receive your protein from poultry or game, fish, or second-class sources. Healthy detox protein choices include chicken, turkey, and game birds such as guinea fowl and partridge.

Talking (and eating) turkey

Turkey is a good detox choice because it contains less saturated fat than any meat other than liver. Turkey is also a good source of the amino acid tryptophan, needed by the brain to manufacture serotonin, a chemical mood mediator.

You can perk up your spirits during detox, should they fall slightly, with a healthy turkey dish, boosting your serotonin level and increasing your feeling of well-being. Serotonin combats any tendency you may have to clinical depression and prolonged attacks of low mood.

Turkey is also rich in zinc, which stabilises blood sugar levels, helps small cuts and abrasions to heal, and maintains the health of the prostate gland (non-cancerous enlargement of this male gland can impede urine flow, and therefore the excretion of toxins and other water-soluble waste matter).

Taming wild fowl and game

Remember to remove the skin of poultry and game birds to reduce your intake of saturated fats. It is also healthier to casserole, poach or microwave suitable meat to avoid using additional cooking fat or oil. Poultry, fowl, and game are all valuable protein sources, and pretty fat-free if you avoid the skin (*and* avoid fat during cooking, of course!)

Chicken is a popular meat and is an excellent source of low-fat protein. Chicken gives you the amino acid tryptophan which provides many essential actions, including the production of the brain-mood chemical serotonin, levels of which are low in depressed people. Chicken is also a good source of B vitamins, especially niacin, which combats cancerous cell change and helps to protect the brain from age-related decline, including Alzheimer's disease. Vitamin B6 (pyridoxine) works with niacin to boost energy levels. Chicken is also a source of phosphorus, which is needed to assimilate niacin; chicken promotes the metabolism of fats and starches (thereby providing energy), and is also said to lessen arthritic pain and to promote healthy teeth and gums.

Turkey, however, has even more benefits than chicken.

Reeling in fish

Eating fish provides plenty of protein, and oily fish have the added benefit of providing you with omega-3 essential fatty acids.

- ✔ Oily fish include mackerel, herrings, tuna, sardines, and salmon.
- ✔ Non-oily fish include plaice, haddock, whiting, cod, coley, and monkfish.
- ✔ Prawns and other shellfish are often shunned by nutritionists for their cholesterol content, but this is in fact very low. Just don't eat them in vast quantities or more than once or twice a week.

More protein sources

Fish and poultry aren't the only source of protein, which is good news for vegetarians. Beans are a good protein source too.

Supping on soya

You may already enjoy tofu (compressed soya bean curd), soy sauce, miso soup (made from fermented soya beans), and soya-based dairy substitutes such as milk, yoghurt, and ice cream or other desserts.

Tofu – curd made from soya bean milk is an excellent source of protein, including tryptophan amino acid, and is rich in omega-3 fatty acids, calcium, magnesium, phosphorus, copper, iron, manganese, and selenium. Recent research has shown that regular intakes of soya, including tofu, can lower total cholesterol by up to 30 per cent and the dangerous type (LDL) by between 35 and 40 per cent. It also reduces triglyceride levels and the blood's tendency to form dangerous clots (thrombosis.) Tofu also contains phyto-oestrogens, especially the isoflavones genistein and diadzein, which act as extrmely weak oestrogens, relieving menopausal symptoms such as hot flushes and sweats, and the tendency to develop osteoporosis. (Many forms of tofu are also calcium-enriched, increasing the protection against this bone-thinning disease.)

All soya and soy products are derived from the soya bean. Soya is a great source of protein, besides supplying fibre, calcium, and isoflavones. These isoflavones, known as phytoestrogens, are anti-oxidants with similar actions to human female hormone oestrogen, and as such offer marked protection against menopausal symptoms, coronary arterial disease, non-cancerous breast disease, fibroids, endometriosis, and certain cancers such as of the prostate gland.

Phytoestrogens also guard against the deterioration in verbal and non-verbal reasoning skills that can occur with age. This may be especially relevant in the case of an older person planning to detox, who fears a degree of memory loss or reasoning ability. Toxins undoubtedly contribute to senile dementia and Alzheimer's disease, making soya products uniquely useful as a protein source.

For optimal effects, you need to eat about 15 grams of soya daily in two equal portions. For example, you can have a soya yoghurt for breakfast, and a drink made with a soya milk replacement at bedtime.

Picking Fruit and Vegetables

Fruit and vegetables are the linchpin of detoxifying your system. They are the main source of vitamins, minerals and trace elements, and they supply fibre and a host of plant constituents called phyto-chemicals such as the phytoestrogens discussed in the preceding 'Supping on soya' section.

Excellent sources of phytoestrogens include avocadoes, bananas, apples, fresh and dried dates, raisins, apricots, figs, prunes, paw-paw, mango, and other tropical fruits.

Many vegetables and fruits also supply potassium, which is needed within cells to balance the sodium present in the blood and tissue fluid. Potassium has a diuretic effect, increasing urine flow and helping to rid the body of excess water and reduce high blood pressure.

Many diuretic drugs prescribed for fluid retention and high blood pressure drive sodium out of the body through the kidneys. They can also drive out a certain amount of potassium, too, which is why the so-called potassium-sparing diuretic drugs – or additional potassium tablets – are often prescribed alongside them to prevent the body from losing too much potassium.

Hesperidin, a bioflavonoid in lemons, grapefruit, and oranges, reduces raised blood pressure, raises the level of healthy choles-terol, and reduces the level of the dangerous variety. Limonene, a constituent of citrus peel, cuts the risks of squamous cell carci-noma of the lungs, skin, and other organs. Ensure that you get your daily intake of citrus fruit nutrients by eating an orange and/or grapefruit each day, and include some peel and pith when juicing. Broccoli and other cruciferous veg (those with cross-shaped flowers), such as Brussels sprouts, cabbage, kale, turnips, and cau-liflower, provide vitamin C, calcium, and magnesium for strong teeth and bones, manganese for powerful muscles and improved memory, and vitamin K, for normal blood clotting. They also cut the risks of cataracts and certain birth defects, and keep the heart and blood vessels in healthy condition.

The benefits of fruit and veg

It's great to know the benefits you can get from eating healthy foods. For example, alfalfa sprouts contain free radical-fighting antioxidants, in particular chlorophyll. They are also high in potas-sium, and contain calcium. Apples and pears are well-known for being high in vitamin C.

See the Appendix for a list of many of the ingredients mentioned in the recipe chapters and the beneficial and detox-related effects each can give you.

Chapter 6

What Not To Eat – and Why

*L*ess really is more when you're detoxing, because the less you eat of toxin-laden foods, the lighter you feel physically and mentally, the fresher and more youthful your appearance, and the better you are able to deal with stress.

In this chapter, I talk about the main foods to ditch during detox and what foods to root out of your cupboard and your eating plan thereafter.

Eschewing 'E' Numbers

Eschewing (rather than chewing!) E number-rich, nutrient-poor convenience foods and similar monstrosities, is the lynchpin of detox. E-numbers refer to the additives such as meat dyes, flavourings and preservatives that manufacturers and commercial processors use in food preparation. Each is designated by a number, preceded by the letter E.

Food likes and dislikes are intensely personal, and most of us fool ourselves about at least some of our choices.

For example, convincing yourself that the meat you buy is quite healthy – provided that you just trim off the fat – is quite easy! Cut the fat off spare ribs by all means, and enjoy them as an occasional treat, but prepare them yourself for the barbecue or oven, with freshly ground (or at any rate unadulterated) spices. Pre-flavoured spare ribs, chops, chicken pieces, and kebabs often appear in lurid colours due to the dye used in their preparation. Food manufacturers bank on our familiarity with the orange-red of real tandoori dishes (for example), to sell us inferior substitutes that they hope we'll never question.

When hunting for E-numbers, inspect labels carefully and discard any foods with artificial flavourings, preservatives, colouring – in fact any additive you do not know to be harmless.

Some additives are okay, such as citric acid, an acidity regulator, and vitamins C (also known as ascorbic acid or ascorbate) and E – both added for their antioxidant action. It's a good idea to buy a small E-number reference book to help you keep up to date with additive usage and trends, and keep it in your bag or pocket when shopping. Write down any unusual ones in your diary or notebook.

In general, vitamins such as those I have just mentioned, all of which are represented by E-numbers when not naturally present in the food concerned, are safe. But if all this sounds too finicky and time-consuming, just avoid everything containing E-numbers and buy good organic produce instead. It's easier and less stressful.

Forgoing False Fats

Fats to avoid are saturated fats such as butter, fatty meat and lard, and *trans fats* – plant oils that start off chock-full of healthy essential fatty acids but are altered into the unhealthy trans form by high-temperature processing techniques. The fats that do you good (although you still need to limit your intake of them) are the omega-3, 6 and 9 fatty acids I discussed in Chapter 5. The need to avoid taking even these in excess is explained by their high calorie content (9 calories per gram as opposed to just 4 calories per gram supplied by protein and carbohydrate). Nutritionists everywhere advise that fats and oils from whatever source, should not contribute more than 20–30% of a person's total calorie intake.

Steering clear of saturated fats

Saturated fats are mainly of animal origin and appear daily on most people's tables. Common examples are butter, lard, the fat around meat, and dripping (that is, the fat that drips of a roasting joint and congeals to a solid substance once the roasting pan is cold). Saturated fats increase the quantity of cholesterol in your bloodstream, especially that of LDL (low density lipoprotein) cholesterol

(– the dangerous sort that readily infiltrates damaged arterial walls and forms deposits or 'plaques', clogging the blood flow).

The two likely outcomes of plaque deposits make for seriously bad news:

✔ The clogging continues until the artery is so bunged-up that only a tiny trickle of oxygen- and nutrient-rich blood can pass through it. Should the organ this artery supplies be the brain, say, or the heart muscle, the oxygen-deprived tissue starts to show signs of dysfunction, giving rise, perhaps, to a mini-stroke in the brain or *angina* (heart pain due to lack of oxygen).

✔ A blood clot may form on top of plaque within the artery's lining, which then causes a heart attack or stroke, frequently with fatal suddenness.

So you need to cut out butter (or eat it *very* occasionally as a special treat), and use a substitute spread made from polyunsaturated, cold-pressed plant oils. Again, inspect labels. The label may say 'high in polyunsaturates' but you need to check whether trans fats – also called hydrogenated vegetable oils – are lurking in the undergrowth.

Transcending trans fats

Trans fats are the exact opposite of the healthy essential fatty acids (EFAs). While the healthy sort (such as linoleic acid, found in sunflower, safflower, corn, and similar plant oils) have vitamin-like actions necessary for normal cell structure and function, trans fats behave like anti-vitamins. They deplete the body of essential *prostaglandins,* short-lived, hormone-like body chemicals that control many aspects of health including skin metabolism, inflammation (which is essentially a protective mechanism), and male and female reproductive cycles.

 To cut out or limit your intake of these noxious turncoats, you have to ensure that the plant oils with which you cook, and the spreads with which you replace butter, are cold-pressed. *Cold-pressed oils* are not subjected to high temperatures and hydrogenation.

Bottles of extra virgin olive oil often say 'cold-pressed' on the label. Expensive speciality oils such as nut oils, avocado oil, and pumpkin oil (used for dressings and to enhance foods' flavours and nutritional value rather than for cooking) are generally cold-pressed.

It's also a good idea to seek out and stick with a butter substitute made from cold-pressed oils.

 It's always wise to check the label before buying any oil or butter substitute, especially as these foods become more popular and widely available. Look specifically for the words 'cold-pressed'; some manufacturers even go so far as to state on the label that no high temperatures are used in the preparation of the food in question.

 Subject oils to the minimum necessary temperatures when using them for cooking. This helps to ensure that the healthy omega-oils you've taken the trouble to use undergo as little transformation as possible into the unhealthy 'trans' types.

Curtailing Carbohydrates

You need to cut down on carbohydrates during detox for two reasons. Firstly, you want to give your body maximum nourishment as well as rest from its usual digestive slog. Fruit and veg are full of easily absorbed vitamins and minerals, and they make minimal demands on your stomach and bowel. In fact, they actively encourage your bowel to shed its toxic load.

Secondly, even healthy low-GI carbs (refer to Chapter 5) contain a little natural glucose and sugar, and to avoid the risks of peaks and troughs of your blood sugar levels it's wise to cut out possible sources of these nutrients other than the plant foods that are the the mainstay of your detox plan.

The chief carbohydrate foods to avoid are junk snacks and processed foods rich in glucose, refined starches (present in white rice, for instance), and sucrose (sugar), all of which have a high glycaemic index rating. (refer to Chapter 5, which talks about the glycaemic index of foods.) These foods have little or no fibre to slow down the entry of their sugar content into your bloodstream, which means that they send your blood glucose levels soaring, which in turn triggers the release of a lot of insulin. This hormone promptly drives sugar (or glucose as it's known in the body) out of the bloodstream and into tissue cells, whereupon two undesirable things happen:

> ✔ Firstly, the insulin can send your blood glucose level plummeting into your socks, sparking symptoms of hypoglycaemia (low blood sugar).These symptoms include shakiness, sweating, weakness, nausea, and a thumping pulse and heart beat. No wonder that many first-time sufferers fear that they are having a coronary or a panic attack.

✔ Secondly, habitually raised insulin levels, triggered by eating sugary snacks and refined starchy products, are linked to obesity, diabetes, and increased risks of developing heart disease or a stroke.

Sweetening without sugar

Glycaemic index ratings compare relevant foods to glucose, which has a rating of 100. Maltose (the sugar into which the digestive system breaks down simple starches) is also rated 100. Honey is slightly healthier, with a G.I. rating of 80, and sucrose is rated at 60. Fructose, found in fruit, has a G.I. rating of 20.

You can satisfy a sweet tooth by gradually reducing your intake of refined sugars and replacing them with the natural sugars present in fruits. A piece of fruit is a healthy alternative to a chocolate bar, just as a glass of fruit juice diluted with water is to a can of fizzy pop. It takes about four weeks until you find the sweet foods you once craved too sweet for comfort.

If you're really serious about cutting back on sweet foods, avoid sugar substitutes. Although they do not affect your blood glucose level, neither do they help you lose your taste for sweets.

Realising white isn't so nice

While you're detoxing – and after – discard refined grains and their products such as white bread (cakes, biscuits, and so on), as well as white rice and pasta in favour of the wholegrain, full-fibre alternatives that release their natural sugars slowly.

Be wary, too, of made-up, pre-packaged meals consisting of flavoured noodles, rice, couscous and similar grains as they will surely contain refined cereals and grains, saturated fat, sugar, and artificial additives.

Shaking Off Salt

It can be as hard, or harder, to cut down on salt than on sugar. If you have always added this condiment when cooking potatoes and other veg, food cooked without it can be miserably bland.

Salt supplies sodium, which is known to increase the risks of suffering from high blood pressure for some people. It also aggravates the problem of fluid retention, which causes bloating and weight gain, and the more salt you take on board, the harder your kidneys are obliged to work. You do need to reduce your salt intake if you tend to retain fluids, and very probably if you suffer from high blood pressure (sodium aggravates hypertension in some sufferers, and has no effect on others – it all depends whether you are susceptible to its effects or not.) Even if your personal health issues don't dictate salt reduction, nutritionists are undoubtedly right in advising us as a nation to consume less sodium. The job of excreting it falls to the kidneys and can overtax them over the long term.

You can cut back on salt by avoiding snacks such as crisps, salted nuts, savoury popcorn, and many processed snacks and meals. Choose plain nuts and crispy (unsalted!) baked potato skins instead, and substitute table and cooking salt with the reduced sodium variety.

You can also grow accustomed to 'saltlessness' by doctoring vegetables, eggs, meat, and other savouries with fresh or dried herbs, condiments, and spices. Here are some suggestions:

- ✔ Add a little English mustard to boiled or mashed potatoes just before serving.
- ✔ Use garlic for potatoes, spinach, peas, beans, and other pulses.
- ✔ Sprinkle caraway seeds on cabbage and spring greens.
- ✔ Try low sodium tomato ketchup or salsa with cauliflower.
- ✔ Spice up root vegetables with nutmeg or cinnamon.
- ✔ Use low-sodium soy sauce in practically everything.

Perk up vegetables by mixing in a little grated, low-fat cheese; vinegar – especially cider or balsamic; or cherry tomatoes or peppers stir-fried till soft with a little garlic and chopped onion.

Deserting Dairy

Full-fat dairy foods are a no-no. However, dairy products contain a range of vital nutrients including calcium, essential for strong bones and teeth. Low-fat dairy contains the full complement of calcium, and you need to avoid full-cream milk, cheese, and similar foods, using skimmed or semi-skimmed alternatives.

You are strongly advised to reduce your intake of dairy products during detox, because you need to cut down the range of foods you put into your body during a detox. Detox emphasises eating and drinking fruit and vegetables and their juices. Dairy products also have a mucus-producing effect (although this is less true of goat's milk than of cow's milk). Your body is already trying to throw off mucus from your gut, nose, throat, and lungs once the detox process gets underway, and you don't want to add to its burden by making it produce extra mucus!

You also need to remain as healthy as possible during detox; and it's a fact that many people are unable to tolerate lactose (milk sugar). This digestive disorder, known as lactose intolerance, generally makes itself apparent in infancy or childhood. If this applies to you, you may not have eaten dairy foods for years!

 While real lactose intolerance means that you will probably always have to avoid cow's milk, you may find that you can take goat's milk products quite safely. It's a matter of suck it and see! But over the past ten years, the goat's milk industry (like the animals themselves!) has progressed by leaps and bounds, becoming far more widely available to an ever-growing demand. Goat's milk and yoghurt are delicious, and you may be missing out on great food and drink pleasure – and a healthy nutrient source! – by not giving them a try.

If you really have to/wish to avoid all animal milk, then you should try (or may already be familiar with) such soya milk alternatives as bread spread, smoothies, yoghurt, and cheese. Soy products have also improved beyond recognition recently, and now come in a wide range.

Going Easy on Grapefruit

Grapefruit juice can slow the action of the cleansing phase of detox, so it's best to avoid this fruit while following a detox programme.

The bioflavonoid, narangin, found originally in oranges (from the Sanskrit word Naranj meaning orange, and one of the oldest words known) interferes with one of the liver enzymes of the cytochrome P 450 series, which you may have heard of because they are important in processing many prescribed drugs. (Patients taking medications such as cyclosporine, the cholesterol-lowering statins, Plendil, Seldane, and Propulsid, are warned to stay off grapefruit juice until their course is finished.)

The cytochrome P 450 enzymes work round the clock to neutralise and get rid of toxins, and they are particularly hard pushed when coping with all the extra toxins released during detox. The last thing you need is something interfering with their efficiency, which is why you need to postpone quaffing grapefruit juice until your detox is complete. All citrus fruit contain a certain amount of narangin, largely in their pith (– the white cheesy part below the skin); but grapefruit alone contain enough narangin to have a metabolic effect.

Part III
Detoxing Your Lifestyle

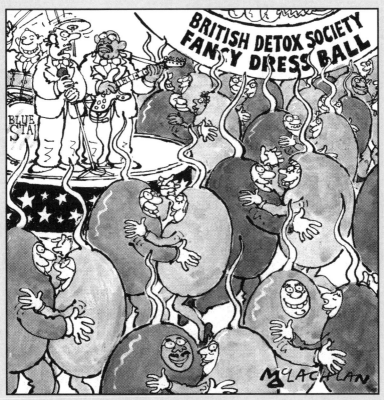

"It's amazing — Everyone this year has come as a bean sprout."

In this part . . .

*H*ere I tell you how to detox your lifestyle and why it is so desirable to do so. In Chapter 7 I talk about toxic habits (such as smoking and drinking large amounts of alcohol) and help you to decide how to eliminate them.

In Chapter 8 I explain how and why stress generates toxic effects within your body. I talk about simple and natural ways to combat the effects of prolonged stress on your immune system.

Chapter 9 is about relaxation, a powerful antidote to both stress and its adverse effects on mind and body. I suggest a number of ways in which you can introduce relaxation into your life, and derive as much benefit as possible from the method of your choice.

Chapter 7

Detoxing Your Lifestyle

● ●

In This Chapter

▶ Banning the booze

▶ Fighting the fags

▶ Conquering the caffeine habit

▶ Downsizing on drugs

● ●

*T*his chapter is about detoxing your lifestyle of unhealthy habits. Chapters 5 and 6 tell you which foods to eat and which to avoid during your detox programme. You also need to cut out alcohol, cigarettes and caffeine, and all but essential medicines during a detox and as part of a healthy lifestyle. This chapter gives you hints and helps to knock these toxins out of your life.

Avoiding Alcohol

Clearly, because breaking down alcohol produces toxins in your body, you have to remain teetotal during detox. To encourage you to do this, I include a few lines about the ill effects of both heavy and binge drinking as well as advice on how to quit drinking altogether.

Realising how heavy is heavy

What constitutes 'heavy' drinking is, to an extent, objective. A precise definition in terms of pints of beer or glasses of wine is not possible. Essentially, however, heavy drinking means drinking significantly more alcohol every week than the Government's safe drinking guidelines advise. The guidelines recommend a maximum of 14 units a week for women, and 21 units for men. One unit equals 100 millilitres (4 fluid ounces) of standard strength wine, 250 millilitres (half a pint) of standard strength lager or beer, a schooner of sherry, vermouth or other fortified wine, or a single 'pub' shot of spirits (with or without a mixer).

The safety guidelines also advise regular drinkers to have at least two alcohol-free days every week, and to spread the rest of their quota over the remaining days.

Several factors influence your ability to metabolise alcohol including

✔ The state of your liver. Your liver has to be fighting-fit to handle the toxins created when breaking down the alcohol.

✔ Your age. Children and teenagers are more readily affected by relatively small quantities. This is because youngsters are smaller than adults, with relatively immature livers and kidneys. A pint of ale, for example, produces a higher blood alcohol concentration in a six-year-old boy weighing 4 stone (because there's far less blood to dilute it) than in a twenty-six-year-old man weighing 11 stone. An adult's liver, moreover, is likely to have handled alcohol and many other toxins over the years, while that of a child is unaccustomed to dealing with such a greatly increased toxin load.

✔ Your gender and the amount of surplus fat you are carrying. You see, alcohol is soluble in water but not in fat; women on the whole are not only lighter than men but they also have more body fat, which means that less blood exists to 'dilute' the alcohol as they drink it. If you're a woman, your blood alcohol concentration may well be higher than that of your male partner, and the effects of drinking – both good and bad – are more pronounced.

Your response may be 'Unfair, or what?' but this is a gender discrepancy against which feminism is utterly powerless!

Being dictated to regarding not only how much alcohol you should drink but also how and when to drink it can feel irritating, but the advice stems from huge scientific studies into alcohol's effects on thousands of men and women and, to remain healthy, you must stick to the guidelines.

Saying no to alcohol

Cut out alcohol by saying 'No'. This may sound brutal when applied to a supreme pleasure (which many regular imbibers swear drinking is), but 'No' is the only way. If you are really serious about detoxing, and long for the health boost it can bring, you have, to coin a pun, no half measures.

Beware of binge drinking

If you are one of the many habitual binge drinkers you may be blissfully unaware of your habit's life-threatening dangers. When you binge-drink, you take on board a whole splurge of alcohol – far more than you usually drink – 'all in one go', by which I mean over the course of an evening, a day or even longer.

Binge drinking, while always perilous, is also to a degree objective: a football fan may down twelve pints of lager with Bacardi chasers to celebrate his team's victory, compared to his 'normal' consumption of just six to seven pints a night. If you're a woman on a girls' night out, perhaps you get through a couple of bottles of wine during the evening, or three or four cocktails and half a dozen or so alcopops.

The social dangers of binge drinking such as the increased risk of rape, mugging, or assault, appear in the press daily, and I am not going to go into them here. From the health point-of-view, however, you are overloading your liver with a massive dose of toxins, which in turn triggers a huge rise in blood pressure. *This rise happens whether or not you usually suffer from high blood pressure.* While you're bingeing, and for several hours afterwards as your liver and kidneys struggle to deal with the toxic overload, this rise in blood pressure greatly increases your risks of a heart attack or stroke.

Also, perhaps unfairly, you cannot reduce the ill effects of bingeing by saving up your weekly quota of units for a big night out, and staying off alcohol for the rest of the week.

Bingeing is a potentially deadly game and, if you go in for it, knowing the risks can make your prospective detox even more attractive.

Saying no to others

Passing up the pint after work or your usual weekend pub crawl with the gang can be a problem unless your fellow drinkers have your welfare very much at heart (unlikely, perhaps, but not impossible). They may not want to join you in detoxing, but real friends will certainly respect your wish to accomplish something quite hard (if you're a heavy drinker) and refrain from offering you booze, or insisting you accompany them to the pub or bar.

Go drinking with your friends by all means if you've a will of iron, or drink very little normally. But an orange juice or mineral water is highly unlikely to satisfy you when you're surrounded by merry drinking pals, if alcohol is a real temptation.

Saying no to yourself

Saying no to yourself can prove even more difficult! But here are some suggestions to get you going:

✔ **Chuck out the alcohol.** Rid your home and office of all stores of alcohol before and during your detox.

✔ **Stock up with soft drinks that you like.** You don't have to 'go without' during an alcohol holiday, simply substitute B for A. If you like a strong drink that takes the breath away, try tomato juice with Worcestershire or Tabasco sauce. If girly drinks are more your thing, try sparkling mineral water over ice, add some crushed strawberries or raspberries and drink it through a straw.

✔ **Concentrate on the positive.** Don't dwell on missing alcohol but on what you hope to gain from going without it while detoxing. Write down three benefits, being as specific and upbeat as you can. 'I don't want to suffer from hangovers' or 'I want to be healthier', are both no-nos. More effective alcohol-abstention detox goals may include, 'I'm cleansing my liver and giving it a new lease of life', or 'I can just *feel* my body organs and skin benefiting from a holiday from alcohol.'

✔ **Line up a strategy for emergencies.** It doesn't matter much what your strategy is. Tom Bombadil in *The Lord of the Rings* taught the hobbits a song to sing when in danger, and they used it to call him to their rescue when ensnared by the Barrow Wight. Whatever you choose, make it intensely personal to yourself, and therefore powerfully meaningful.

Say a short prayer, recite lines of a much-loved poem, mentally hum a bar or two of a favourite melody or, more prosaically, visualise your next delicious detox snack or meal like mad!

You can use any diversionary tactic you like, providing it deflects your attention and desire away from the bottle or glass.

For instance, some water buffs, who find this element evocative and satisfying on more than one level, quaff a glass of plain water when pressurised to drink, or, if the occasion permits, take a long hot or cold shower, and sip ice-cold mineral water afterwards.

Stopping Smoking

As happens when you are withdrawing from any addictive substance, symptoms of irritation, low mood, poor sleep, and acute cravings can develop. So, unless you are an exceptionally strong-willed person with mountains of stamina and a determination of tempered steel, you are far better off cutting down and finally stopping your smoking habit *before* starting your detox.

Please try not to postpone your detox indefinitely on the grounds that you need to stop smoking first! The human mind has a genius for coming up with excellent 'excuses' to avoid challenging life changes. You are better off attempting a detox plan even if you really can't cut out cigarettes altogether than not detoxing at all.

Knowing why you smoke

Smoking is so politically incorrect these days that very few smokers come up with a straight answer when asked why they smoke. Many say they hate cigarettes and would love never to buy another packet. Others claim that they've stopped smoking in the past, but accepted one at a party in a moment of abstraction, and 'That was it!' Yet others blame their habit on stress at work, a recent bereavement, a troubled partnership, or even Christmas, having their mother-in-law to stay, or the family dog! Very few people cut to the chase, and admit freely, 'I smoke because I like it!'

Looking at cigarettes' attraction

As you intend quitting, it helps to work out what smoking actually does for you, because then you can find healthy substitutes. All smokers and ex-smokers recognise the secret comfort of a cigarette packet in their pocket or handbag ('The one friend who *won't* let me down'). Then there's the sheer enjoyment of lighting up (personal rituals are important to most of us), inhaling a lungful of smoke, and calming the cravings or irritable mood that have been giving you hassle.

Peering into cigarettes' (very) dark side

Tobacco smoke contains more than 300 chemicals, of which nicotine is the key figure. Nicotine is more addictive than heroin and so lethal that the quantity in one packet of 20 ciggies would kill you stone dead if you swallowed it. Next to alcohol, nicotine is the most duplicitous 'mate' on earth.

Yes, it can calm you down when you're overwrought, subdue hunger pangs by raising your blood glucose level, and perk you up when you're driving or studying, or after a heavy meal. At the same time, however, nicotine encourages clogging of the arteries both to the heart (the coronaries) and to other vital organs.

In addition, up to 20 of the other chemicals in cigarette smoke are known to cause cancer, particularly of the lungs, and increase the risks of malignancy in many other organs such as the mouth, throat, oesophagus, stomach, bowel, cervix, and breast.

Smoking is also responsible for a great deal of non-cancerous lung damage such as emphysema and other forms of chronic obstructive airways disease (COAD). Watching blue-lipped victims gasping into their oxygen masks, unable even to reach their own bathrooms or bedrooms unaided, soon puts the delights of smoking into clear perspective.

Planning healthy substitutes

Forward planning can make all the difference to your chances of successfully quitting smoking. Decide the day on which you intend quitting, and label it Q day in your diary or on a calendar (perhaps one to three weeks ahead). Think about it often, remember what a great gift you'll be giving yourself, and look forward to the opportunity to improve your health.

First of all, though, look to your diet to supply the 'benefits' that smoking supplies.

Choosing nutrition over cigarettes

Root out and toss away all junk food! Now is not the time to compensate for cigarette withdrawal with high-sugar, high-fat snacks and takeaways. Think whole, fresh, organic . . . and turn to the following:

- ✔ Eat low-G.I. carbohydrates, which are full of fibre, and release glucose slowly into your bloodstream. Low-G.I. foods maintain your blood glucose level within normal limits and reduce the risks of hunger pangs, exhaustion, and irritability. Wholegrains, vegetables and many fruits are low-G.I., and can take the place of all sugar and refined foods that upset your glucose level.

- ✔ Eat protein twice or three times daily, to supply essential amino acids including tryptophan, which has a direct lifting effect on mood, as well as improving pain thresholds and sleep. Fish, lean white meat and game, eggs, soya, and combinations of beans, lentils, grains, and nuts are all fine choices. Rich sources of tryptophan include turkey, chicken breast, cod, shrimps, soya, cottage cheese, and Brazil nuts.

- ✔ Avoid saturated animal fats and hydrogenated plant oils. You can obtain oils and fats from oily fish (three portions a week), cold-pressed vegetable oils, nuts, and seeds. If you cannot eat fish, take fish oil supplements instead.

- ✔ Eat little and often to maximise digestion and further aid normal blood glucose levels. Combine carbohydrates with protein foods when you can, to optimise the passage of essential amino acids into the brain.

✔ Take lecithin as a supplement. Lecithin is a naturally occurring fat is rich in phospholipids, which biochemists and doctors have known about for many decades but which have now been found to improve the mood and reduce the risks of dementia. Egg yolks are rich in phospholipids, but lecithin can be bought in granule or capsule form. You need around five grams of lecithin daily, or half this quantity if your lecithin supplement is the 'high-PC' variety, rich in phosphatidyl choline.

✔ Reduce nicotine cravings with supplements of oat straw (Avena sativa) and sunflower seeds. Follow the label advice for the oat straw supplement, or chew a medium-sized handful of sunflower seeds 3–4 times a day or whenever the cravings bother you.

✔ Drink lots of water (perhaps 10–12 glasses a day as opposed to your now-normal 8–10 glasses) to enable your kidneys to rinse smoking by-products out of your bloodstream.

Stress-busting while you quit

Take up a simple relaxation technique and practice it while preparing to quit smoking. You'll find it an invaluable tool for coping with stress. Chapter 8 talks about stress. Relaxation methods are explained in Chapter 9.

Taking the final steps to quitting

Here are the steps to follow in quitting smoking. And, above all, make sure that you dwell on your success, and the improved health and life expectancy that will result. Perhaps you have failed to quit in the past; but since when was past failure a reliable indicator of the future?

✔ Gradually reduce the number of cigarettes you smoke daily, starting with those that you are least likely to miss.

✔ On Quit Day, remove temptation by throwing away all cigarettes, empty packets, lighters and matches, and give away your ashtrays. Concentrate on getting through each day, aided by frequent sips of water, or fruit or vegetable juice, or chewing some sugar-free gum, or sucking sugar-free sweets.

✔ When the urge to smoke strikes, say to yourself, 'I really can't be bothered. All that hassle for the sake of giving myself cancer. It really isn't worth it!'

✔ Improve the health of your lungs and take advantage of extra doses of oxygen by going outside, or to an open window, and taking 9–10 slow deep breaths, holding each when your lungs are full, and then slowly exhaling. Repeat four to five times a day at least.

✔ Visualise your lungs slowly turning from brown, toxin-ridden organs into healthy, pink, efficient ones.

✔ Avoid the company of friends, colleagues and relatives who smoke, or at least ask them not to do so around you.

✔ Clean your teeth with a strongly-flavoured toothpaste, the taste of which you like, and rinse your mouth out with a flavoured mouthwash several times a day.

✔ Use an essential oil product called Nicobrevin to reduce the cravings.

✔ Eat healthy, low-G.I. carbohydrates (see Chapter 5, What To Eat and Why), to gently activate your insulin to deal with the smoothly rising blood sugar level triggered by the carbs. Insulin activity also helps to combat nicotine cravings. This may account for the craving for sweet snacks, which many recently-quit smokers experience (although high-G.I. foods containing refined sugar and white flour are not the answer because they activate insulin in an unhealthy manner).

Quitting Caffeine

Coffee reached Europe from the Middle East during the seventeenth century and, together with tea, it accounts for about 98 per cent of worldwide caffeine consumption. We drink coffee because it's delicious, fashionable, and a great booster of energy and mood. Nowadays, students and others preparing for exams are less likely to burn the midnight oil than they are to make frequent cups of coffee, or strong tea, by day and by night.

A cup of strong tea contains approximately the same amount of caffeine as a weak cup of coffee and its tannin content can interfere with the absorption of minerals and trace elements. Many people get further caffeine fixes from cola drinks.

Calculating caffeine's 'desirable' effects

Caffeine's effect on the brain is to increase the levels of two neurotransmitters – adrenaline and dopamine. As caffeine hits your bloodstream, you feel buoyant, alert and ready to plough through masses of paperwork at a time when non-coffee drinkers are propping their eyelids open with matchsticks – during the middle of the afternoon, in a warm office, for instance, or after a heavy lunch.

Also in caffeine's favour is the speed at which your body eliminates it. After a fix, caffeine takes between thirty minutes and an hour to reach its peak concentration in the blood, after which this miscreant is handed over to the liver. This excretory organ handles caffeine so efficiently that the level in the bloodstream is reduced to half the peak concentration after only four to six hours.

Adding up caffeine's negatives

Caffeine is extremely addictive, meaning that you require more and more of it to achieve the same result. Withdrawal symptoms, which you may or may not have experienced so far, include headaches, a drop in mood, fatigue, poor concentration, and sleepiness.

Caffeine also raises the blood glucose and cholesterol levels and can irritate an acid stomach, causing heartburn. (Raising blood glucose is temporarily beneficial, but as caffeine is excreted from the body, the blood glucose level of this nutrient can plummet quickly, leaving you weak and shaky).

Like other stimulants, caffeine can overtax the adrenal glands that manufacture the stress hormones adrenaline and noradrenaline. Caffeine also interferes with sleep, can cause an irritable mood and, in some people, increases the risks of a coronary (heart attack). Caffeine is also a diuretic, boosting the formation of urine, which in turn can lead to dehydration.

 You need to cut out caffeine during detox so, if you drink a lot of tea, coffee or cola you should start cutting down, making weaker cups, and gradually substituting it with water, fruit or vegetable juice in the fortnight before your detox programme starts.

You may also find yerba maté (pronounced ma-tay) tea useful when cutting out caffeine. It contains a small quantity of caffeine, along with theophylline and theobromine, which increase alertness and concentration, combat drowsiness, and can give a feeling of physical and mental well-being. Apparently, however, yerba maté does not interfere with sleep, produce addiction or bludgeon the adrenal glands as do the more usual caffeine drinks. In fact, it can actually improve sleep disturbance, giving rise to a more refreshing rest.

Also in contrast to coffee, tea, and cola, yerba maté is a popular indigestion remedy. It also helps the bowel excrete toxins by softening hard stools, and encouraging the elimination of waste through both the gut and kidneys.

Ditching Inessential Drugs

Ditching drugs seems a sound idea, but how can you decide which drugs to take and which to put to one side? Frankly, telling your GP that you will not be needing your monthly prescription for, say, your blood pressure medication because you'll be detoxing, is extremely unlikely to evoke a sympathetic response.

Therefore, *if* you are tempted to discard regularly prescribed medication, at least discuss the implications with your doctor first and listen impartially to his or her views (and if you dislike or distrust him or her, make sure that you seek a second opinion). You needn't even mention your detox plans, because if you can safely leave off medication for a fortnight (say) before and during a detox programme, the question arises as to whether you actually need the drug at all.

Recognising essential medication

Every effort is made nowadays to accommodate patients' wishes and views regarding their treatment, even when they cannot possibly be expected to understand the full implications of their disorder. Far removed from arrogance, this is a simple statement of fact. A doctor cannot make patients take their medicines and (contrary to the popular misconception that doctors adore playing God), I have never yet met a medic who would wish to do so. (They also have the ever-strengthening tentacles of compensation culture to consider. . . .)

Undeniably, though, many conditions scream out loud for professional monitoring and treatment, and it can be little short of heartbreaking to listen to patients decline antihypertensive drugs to control their blood pressure (for example), insulin or blood glucose-lowering agents for their diabetes, antidepressants for clinical depression, or injections or tablets to relieve schizophrenia or other psychotic illnesses.

Basically, what you can safely spurn and what you need to take regularly is a matter of common sense. Common conditions for which you should continue treatment on your doctor's advice even during detox include angina and other symptoms of heart disease, high blood pressure, diabetes, cancer, clinical depression, schizophrenia and other psychotic illnesses, asthma, chronic obstructive airways disease (COAD), acute disorders such as appendicitis, gallbladder inflammation, meningitis, childhood (and adult) infectious illnesses, and blood disorders including all forms of anaemia.

Re-evaluating nonessential medication

Sometimes – make that often – pain killers containing codeine and stronger compounds such as diazepam and Valium, which combat anxiety and panic attacks, and hypnotics that relieve insomnia such as temazepam or temaze, are inappropriately prescribed. By this, I mean they are given when a non-addictive alternative (or no medication at all) would have been preferable, or given out as repeat prescriptions long after the patient's need for them has ceased.

Occasionally, of course, patients are so loath to be weaned off these drugs, that they become just a tad difficult during a consultation. Lamentably, the pressurised doctor finds it simpler to issue the prescription than to continue to argue the toss with the patient. This is *not* good medicine, but its development is closely related to the ten-minute consultation time doctors and patients are now allotted in which to commune with one another, and to the erosion of the mutual respect patient and doctor once felt.

You know whether you take pain killers and/or anxiety/relaxant drugs because you seriously need them or not. If you doubt that you need a medication any longer, I urge you to see your GP and talk the matter over. You can, with help, stop taking the most addictive substances, and your detox will be all the more beneficial if you are to do so.

Chapter 8

Overcoming Stress

*N*early everyone suffers from the twenty-first century scourge of stress, and you would doubtless love to reduce the amount you meet daily. But what has stress to do with detox?

Stress – the sort that makes you tense and anxious, as opposed to the sort that excites you – attacks your body in a similar way to chemical and environmental toxins. It encourages the formation of *free radicals,* those supercharged oxygen particles that attack the immune system, and is a major trigger for many major diseases including cancer, high blood pressure, heart and blood-vessel disorders, diabetes, and obesity.

You need to reduce or counteract stress if you're to benefit fully from detox and recharge your immune system and energy levels.

Defining Stress

Stress is the effect on your body of challenging situations that your mind registers as dangerous in themselves (such as walking along a cliff edge), or threatening to your peace of mind and ultimate health (such as a row with your nearest and dearest).

Stress stimulates the adrenal glands, which pour adrenaline into your circulation – sometimes as much as 300 times your normal level. If you can't give vent to your feelings with some vigorous physical action, then symptoms such as tense muscles, a racing pulse, and butterflies in your stomach result.

Muscular aches and pains, tension headaches and migraines, diarrhoea or constipation, irritable bladder, insomnia, and eating disorders are all linked to ongoing negative stress, as are premature ageing, anxiety and depression, poor concentration and memory, and malfunctioning liver and gut (among other organs).

Stressful situations *in themselves* are neither harmful nor beneficial; how you perceive them and handle them, is.

To identify your personal sources of stress, called *stressors,* you have to understand a little about stress and how to distinguish between the damaging sort and the healthy sort.

Many forms of stress are actually quite positive: Skydiving, skiing, horse riding, absailing, and the scariest ride at a fair or circus all provide an adrenaline buzz – if you like that sort of thing! Other stimulating challenges include sitting an exam, performing karaoke, giving a speech, watching a horror film, and asking a celebrity for an autograph.

Harmful stress, by contrast, comprises all the little niggles that, day after day, erode your defences, exhaust you and wear you down. Transport problems, minor ailments, disturbed sleep, crabby neighbours, and boring work all take their toll.

Worst of all is the stress over which you have (or believe that you have) no control. Being bullied or made redundant, losing money or reputation, getting divorced, suffering a bereavement, receiving a diagnosis of cancer or other serious illness in yourself or a loved one can leave you immobilised with fear and a sitting duck for stress's damaging effects.

Identifying Your Stressors

Some negative factors become so familiar, you may not see than as sources of stress at all. Your partner's night-time snores may barely register in your conscious mind, but they still interfere with your sleep. Sarcastic comments from a colleague may seem like water off a duck's back to you, but they can still damage you emotionally. You may accept cheeky, disobedient children as par for the course of parenthood but you may be unaware of the rage boiling away deep inside you.

Life is never a bowl of cherries, and you face and deal with challenges and obstacles daily. But look more closely at your home life, work environment, family relationships, social life, health, personal partnership, and you can surely identify some significant personal stressors.

Signs of Stress

Here are a few of the 'inner feelings' stress may cause:

- ✔ Feeling tense inside, as though a coiled spring is about to become unleashed

- ✔ Getting angry quickly in certain situations, where you feel you want to shout, scream, swear, or throw things

- ✔ Feeling really low, lacking in energy and depressed between experiences of acute tension

- ✔ Feeling extremes of negative emotion such as hatred, resentment, jealousy, vengefulness that are out of proportion to the situation or people involved.

Effects of stress on your mental functions can include:

- ✔ Poor concentration

- ✔ Poor short-term memory where you may repeat tasks or ask questions several times over without realising it or fail to retain simple directions, instructions or information

- ✔ Poor cognitive (reasoning) ability where you find yourself unable to complete tasks which have never before troubled you, such as mental arithmetic, writing shopping lists or letters, performing your usual tasks at home or at work

- ✔ Quickly losing your self-esteem and confidence because of your reduced coping powers.

Both intellectual and emotional changes can be due to depressive illness, early dementia and other illnesses, so check with your GP if you are in doubt. However, depression and dementia tend to develop relatively slowly over a longer period than stress effects, and your doctor will look for other signs and symptoms to help identify the underlying cause.

Physical indicators of stressors at work can include:

- ✔ Tense, aching muscles

- ✔ Tension headaches (or migraine attacks if you're a sufferer)

- ✔ Worsening PMT or menopausal symptoms such as feeling uncomfortable, flushing, sweating, irritability, poor skin and complexion

- ✔ Poor sleep

- ✔ Altered appetite – you're right off your food or tempted to comfort eat

✔ Bouts of nausea, sickness, diarrhoea, or frequent urination

✔ Pounding heart, palpitations (awareness of your heart thumping), rapid pulse, sweating heavily (when not menopausal or overheated).

A little quiet observation and thought soon reveals the presence of significant, ongoing problems in typically stressful situations as the following sections demonstrate.

Fussing with your family

Perhaps it's no coincidence that family springs to most people's mind when stress triggers are mentioned. I cannot even begin to go into the complexities that often make family members the people you 'cannot live with, and cannot live without'. Like a partner's snoring, you get used to the wallpaper of your nearest and dearest's conversation and behaviour, to the point of barely registering their nuisance value (or, often, their great points).

Here's some things to watch for if you think your family is causing you stress:

✔ Feeling angry and irritable with some family members most of the time

✔ Being annoyed by everything they do

✔ Complaining at them or nagging them more than usual, without being able to stop yourself.

Jousting at your job

The four most common reasons people give for disliking their job are:

✔ It asks too much or too little of them.

✔ It bores them stupid.

✔ It underpays them.

✔ It involves contact with non-empathetic, bullying, or otherwise difficult people.

You may know only too well why you get stressed out at work, and what you'd like to do instead. Aside from job availability, one problem is that your work environment, colleagues, and boss eventually become as familiar as your home and family.

Perhaps you even grow a thick skin to shield you from insensitive remarks, poor rewards for your efforts and unhealthy or unaesthetic surroundings. Yet all the while, stress factors are beavering away at your body and emotions, with a possibly unpleasant outcome.

So, how can you tell whether your job is giving you stress? Look at the following and see whether any or all apply:

- ✔ You feel increasingly that you cannot bear to go on with the job.

- ✔ You develop any of the above symptoms given in the family section in a more severe form when going into work or facing a difficult boss or colleague.

- ✔ You spend disproportionate time worrying and feeling bad about work when you're not actually at work.

Letting time get away from you

If you tend to be late for work, appointments and other dates rather than smart, smiling, spruce and half-an-hour early, then your every-day stress is undoubtedly compounded by being grumbled at. Other people (especially the smart, spruce, early birds) find unpunctuality most irritating (as indeed it can be), while remaining in the dark about the stress most late-comers experience.

Habitually late people *are* more stressed. And speaking as one who used always to be late for everything, I can promise you that unpunctuality is generally more wearing than a little forward plan-ning. One reward of being punctual is the right to smile smugly at your colleagues, who (for once) have no grounds for nagging or putting you down.

Many people seem to chase their tails all day, achieving little yet becoming stressed and exhausted in the process. The physical and mental fatigue and the feeling of being constantly harried, often dampens the mood, which, in turn, makes it harder to cope with life's (often unreasonable-seeming) demands. If this applies to you, then maybe you are concentrating on the wrong things.

The thinking behind this suggestion is the *80/20 rule* or *Pareto Principle,* which states that (in general), 80 per cent of your effort produces a mere 20 per cent of results. Meanwhile (you've guessed it!) eighty per cent of results are generated by just twenty per cent of the effort.

Ask yourself whether any (or all) of the following occur when you're preparing to get somewhere on time?

✔ You fuss around and so become late for appointments such as going to work, visiting the hairdresser, seeing your doctor, dentist, or solicitor.

✔ You lie in bed the night before an appointment dreading what you have to do the next day.

✔ You try really hard to organise yourself on time, but *still* find yourself running for the bus or train.

Stressors tend to work collectively rather than singly. Any of the above may be knock-on effects of more general stress, and stress related to family, your job and so on. Take time out to consider repairing the underlying problem, such as building bridges with family or colleagues, and reviewing your job options.

Fidgeting about your finances

Personal finances are one of the most stressful factors in life. You may find yourself worrying like mad about increasing debt, while failing to correct the underlying cause.

If you are a gambler, addicted to shopping, or driven to seek retail therapy when your mood is low, you need specialist help *now* and I urge you to seek it from your doctor who will make the appropriate referrals. If you just cannot balance your weekly books, seek guidance from the Citizens' Advice Bureau (www.citizensadvice.org.uk) – it's free, pertinent and the volunteers really care about helping you deal with your problems.

If you think that your finances may be causing you stress, consider whether the following apply to you:

✔ You constantly have money on your mind. You are fretting about how to pay your bills or wondering how to steer clear of tempting shops when you're skint.

✔ You start to feel that you *hate* money because it's dominating your life.

Either of the above can result in poor sleep, lack of appetite, mood swings, fatigue, and can lead to a bout of depression and physical illness.

Taking care of your health

Most of us (including or perhaps especially doctors) worry about our health at some time in our lives. The concerns tend to treble as the years pass, especially if you haven't paid much attention to a healthy lifestyle previously.

Look for the following signs that health anxiety is stressing you:

✔ You find yourself reading more articles about others' health than you used to.

✔ You start worrying about small 'symptoms' – are you developing the disease you've read about?

✔ You lie awake cursing yourself for not having had a mammogram, cervical smear, blood pressure or cholesterol check, or your eyes tested.

✔ You develop signs of stress (see above), which aggravate any symptoms you've noticed and make you even more afraid to visit your GP.

Whatever you do, just *go*! Make the appointment, have the tests, reassure yourself that your fears are groundless, remember the huge contribution to your health being made by a detox. Resolve to be more health-conscious in future (or commence treatment and allay your anxiety this way).

Handling Your Stress

Getting a handle on your stress is essential to, well, *handling* it. By this I mean identifying the worst culprits among your present stressors, and deciding what to do about them.

General advice for handling most types of stress includes writing down the main points that bother you, or, better still, discussing them with an empathic friend or colleague. Decide on a plan A (the activities most likely to help) and also a plan B (essential), which you can keep up your sleeve in case plan A doesn't work.

Make sure that you talk to your doctor if the stress is making you depressed and unable to cope, or you suffer from chronic sleeping problems.

Use detox to take time out for yourself, and combat the harmful effects of stress on your mind and body.

Detox may amplify stress symptoms at first, because your body is deprived of toxic treats and working extra hard to expel toxins. If you drink plenty of water, follow the advice given in Part IV 'Planning your detox' and also the menu and relaxation ideas (plus supplements!), the adverse effects should be minimal.

Resolving conflict

Some conflicts can be sorted out with mutual discussion over a coffee or healthy snack. Others may require that a third party be present for optimal results, acting as a mediator rather like a marriage guidance counsellor helps a couple get equal say and equal listening time when their partnership is threatened.

Before you try professional help try some of the following ideas.

1. **Arrange a time to talk to the person who upsets you.**

   Do this whether they are a close friend, a relative, partner, child or someone at work. It's a good idea to write down the points you need to make so that nervousness does not disrupt your conversation. Don't rehearse your points over and over again. You may find you become obsessive, and you may find that the thoughts will not leave you alone.

2. **Put forward your own views in an unchallenging way.**

   Make sure that you smile in a friendly way when the two of you meet, relaxing beforehand so that your muscles and facial contours look and feel relaxed, then taking a deep breath and leading into what you want to discuss. Try to let the other person know that you can see his or her side of the conflict and acknowledge their right to hold different views. Then speaking gently but firmly, sketch out what exactly has been troubling you.

3. **Really listen to what the other person is saying.**

4. **You will only find listening difficult if you don't normally do it.**

   Practise on a couple of innocuous people in advance of your appointment (let there be some sort of adverse aspect to communicating with them, such as their having an accent you find hard to understand, or an irritating laugh). Smile, relax, and ask them to explain their views on something (even if you've heard it a thousand times before).

5. **Try to reach an agreement on how to improve things from now on.**

   Be willing to compromise and to give. Also be willing to take!

Working through job problems

Before deciding to quit your job, give the following tips a try:

✔ If you like your job apart from the pay, ask for a rise! Asking would be positively stressful, and get your adrenaline levels zooming! If the answer is 'No,' ask how you can enhance your value to the firm, so that pay rise(s) would follow.

✔ If you're overworked and unappreciated (aren't we all!), explain to your manager that you need more time to complete your tasks efficiently. Suggest possible solutions after first discussing any work delegation with any colleagues involved.

✔ If you're being bullied, discuss the matter with a trusted colleague – others may be experiencing similar treatment. If the matter is too big for you to handle alone, speak to the staffing department or your boss.

If you're becoming depressed, overanxious or you cannot sleep, chat to your GP and ask for time off sick. No job, anywhere, is worth having if it gives you a nervous breakdown.

Managing your time

One time-management course I attended advised concentrating on what you mean to achieve, not just upon being busy. You can get so used to daily rituals such as checking internal memos and scanning your e-mail inbox that you do them regardless of their relevance, and kid yourself you've been hard at work. You then feel pressurised and stressed, and are no nearer to completing your task.

This harried, yet unproductive, business can apply to any task – at work, home, with a hobby – that involves performing certain jobs.

To foil this common habit, it helps to choose an occupation – and an individual task – that you enjoy! No work ethic in the world decrees that work – even hard work – needs to be unpleasant. All jobs have their downside and you and/or the team members carry them out willy-nilly. When taking on tasks and a livelihood, consulting your personal tastes as well as your qualifications and skills, makes a great deal of sense.

Also, if you constantly stress out that you're not achieving enough (as many overanxious people do), then redefine your job with your boss to ensure that you share common priorities, or discuss your work approach with others in your field with a view to eliminating unnecessary tasks you may have considered essential.

Keeping a function-food-fluid diary

Try keeping a diary for one week, recording how you spend your work days. Getting it down in writing (or on the screen) helps you achieve two things:

✔ You get a clear picture of where some of your precious time is being wasted (for example chatting, walking about, queuing for coffee).

✔ You identify tasks on which you spend too much time or which don't have any real value for the target in hand.

Also include in your diary how you feel at different times in the day – alert, drowsy, physically tired, working effectively, finding it hard to work at all. Record what you've had to eat and drink that day (and the night before), including the number of glasses of water you remembered to sip throughout. Alertness, concentration, memory and mood can all be adversely affected by dehydration, as can your meal times and food choices (types and amounts of carbohydrate, protein, fruit and vegetables, and so on).

Finally, mark in your diary time spent on exercise. A brisk lunchtime walk or swim can keep you more alert during the afternoon than chatting in the canteen (or your kitchen) over a cup of coffee. Yoga is ideally suited to flexing and strengthening tense, sore muscles, calming the heart and mind, and improving your inner balance and energy levels.

Making a magical, prioritised to-do list

Making a to-do list magically cuts to the chase – or, more precisely, cuts a swathe through the chaotic welter of time-consuming commitments and jobs that stress you out even to think of them. It also gathers together every last thing you need to do in the most constructive and efficient order, starting with the most essential.

You may be surprised how actually defining the tasks at hand and jotting them down in a prioritised list from most crucial to less important, limits their power to cause you anxiety and stress. Follow these steps to create an effective list:

1. **Write down everything you can think of that belongs on your to-do list.**

2. **Break down large jobs into simpler ones.**

   So, 'research next chapter for my book' becomes 'decide headings beforehand' and 'check my Internet connection works properly'.

3. **Read through your list and allocate each entry a number from one to six where one is 'extremely important' and six is 'can wait'.**

   If you end up with too many priority tasks, break them down further into their component parts. Then, rewrite your list in the order your efforts have worked out is best for you.

4. Decide on your time span.

Some jobs by their very nature may take weeks or even months to complete, so make a second list to be completed in a day, say, or a week. For example, you are unlikely to research your new book's chapter in a day unless you abandon every other task to do so. It doesn't matter if really trivial jobs get moved from one list to the next providing you ultimately do them.

5. Pin up your list (or several copies of it) at strategic points where you cannot fail to see it throughout the day.

6. Most importantly – cross jobs off as you finish them!

If you are new to this technique, the satisfaction crossing jobs off your list provides may well astound you!

De-stressing Herbs and Foods

Herbs and foods can help to minimise the toxic effects of stress, or prevent it from developing in the first place. The following subsections tell you about the most effective in each category.

Relaxing with herbal remedies

Many people believe that, being 'natural', herbal remedies are incapable of causing harm. But herbs have to be medically potent to achieve their effects, and excessive amounts can certainly prove harmful. Always buy plant remedies from an established manufacturer or qualified medical herbalist, and take them exactly as directed.

Having said that, tranquillising herbs, unlike their allopathic (orthodox medical) counterparts, are not known to cause dependency or addiction.

Valerian (Valeriana officinalis)

Probably the best-known herb for combating nervous tension and bringing restful sleep, valerian grows wild throughout Europe and the Near East. It has been used for its sedative effects at least since the time of Ancient Greece and Roma, and was described by Hippocrates, the Greek father of Western medicine.

Valerian induces restful sleep through the combined actions of a number of its constituents, but valerenic acid and compounds called iridoids have also been shown in research studies to have sedative properties.

You need to take about 400 to 500 milligrams of the dried roots or stems before bedtime, avoiding alcohol in the evening because it can enhance valerian's actions. Valerian is not known to interact adversely with other remedies or medicines, though some people report mild side effects such as nausea and dizziness.

You can take valerian as a tea, which you make from sachets of the dried herb, or in a product such as 'Quiet Life', which contains valerian, lettuce extract, and other sleep-inducing herbs.

Lemon Balm (Melissa officinalis)

You may already grow lemon balm, a mint-like herb with a most soothing and calming perfume reflecting its therapeutic properties as a nervous tension remedy.

Known for centuries for its stress-relieving actions, lemon balm was also prescribed for students by the sixteenth-century herbalist John Gerard 'to quicken the senses'. More recently, lemon balm has been shown to relieve mild depression as well as anxiety and to improve *secondary memory,* which is the learning, storing and retrieval of information rather than the recollection of daily events.

Lemon balm contains aromatic oils as well as the antioxidants vitamin C and bioflavonoids, which combat toxins and free radicals.

You can make fresh lemon balm leaves into a tea (a handful of leaves to a large cup of boiling water), or take the dried herb in commercially prepared sachets or capsules. Herbal suppliers often combine this lemon-scented herb with valerian in stress-relieving remedies, and the recommended dose is between 300 and 900 milligrams daily in divided doses before meals. For example, you would take, say 100 mg thrice daily if you're taking 300 mg; or 300 mg thrice daily if you're taking 900 mg.

Lemon balm has not been reported to have any adverse effects or interactions with prescribed medicines.

Ginseng (Panax qinquefolium)

You may already have taken ginseng, a herb renowned for its tonic properties for more than 7,000 years. It has an overall balancing effect upon the body, equalising your metabolic rate (speed of burning food fuel) and your energy levels and vitality. Regular users report greater well-being and physical and emotional stamina as well as improved alertness and concentration.

The above benefits make ginseng a fitting herbal supplement to counteract stress, and restore energy and tranquillity sapped by chronic worry. The roots contain the active constituents, and the herb tends to be sold as white ginseng (the air-dried root), or as red (more potent and stimulating), which is prepared by steaming the roots before drying them.

Chinese, Korean, and Asian varieties are available, depending upon the herb's country of origin. To combat stress and its effects, choose the Korean or Chinese type, which acts as a pick-me-up when you're weak from physical and emotional exhaustion.

Alternatively, choose extract supplements of the closely related American ginseng, *Panex quinquefolius*, found in the forests of central and eastern America. Its milder effects and sweeter flavour make it a favourite with stressed people seeking relief from nervous exhaustion, anxiety and insomnia.

The dosage to follow is printed on the package. Follow the directions given, which will vary between products as so many different ginseng products, and so many methods of preparation are available.

Reishi (Ganoderma lucidum)

Reishi is a mushroom, also known as *ling zhi*, grows on the dead and living wood of deciduous trees, and is extensively used in traditional Chinese medicine to treat a wide spectrum of disorders. Prominent among them are such stress-related conditions as nervous exhaustion, insomnia, and emotional outbursts, irritability and mood swings.

Reishi's healing properties, which have been recognised for at least 2,000 years, are believed to help extend the human lifespan, possibly through a beneficial action on the immune defence system. Reishi is used both in the Far East and in the US and Western Europe for its sedative benefits, and is said to be a potent agent against entrenched sleep disturbances.

It improves the flow of the blood in the system (as well as reducing cholesterol and high blood pressure) but, because of this action on the circulation, seek advice from your doctor before taking it if you are also taking anticoagulant medicines such as Warfarin or a daily aspirin.

Take a reishi supplement for no more than four months at a time and give yourself a break of a month or so before starting again. The break is to minimise the risks of side effects but, even if you do not experience any, you are better off taking a break, if only to improve the body's response to the supplement after such a break. Side effects, which have arisen in those who have taken larger-than-prescribed doses of reishi for far longer periods, include an all-over-body itch, dryness in the nose, throat, mouth, and mucous membranes, and nosebleeds.

The suggested dose is three 1 gram capsules, three times daily, totalling 9 grams, but, as with all supplements, buy the product only from an established and recognised manufacturer, and follow the packet directions carefully.

Astragalus (Astragalus membranaceous)

Also known as milk-vetch root or *huang oi*, *astralagus* is a pretty, perennial herb that grows in the wild in China and Mongolia where it can be identified by its hairy leaves and its pale pink and yellow flowers.

Astragalus has a number of beneficial effects upon the immune defence system, which takes a severe battering when you are subjected to prolonged and intense stress. The sum total of effects is said to prolong the human lifespan. The effects of specific relevance to detox and stress include the relief of fatigue and chronic fatigue syndrome, and protection from coughs, colds, and other minor infectious illnesses, which frequently affect you when you are feeling debilitated.

Astragalus has no recorded side effects, but consult your doctor before taking this supplement if you are taking antiviral medication such as acyclovir (prescribed for *herpes* infections), because *astragalus* can exaggerate its effects. The same advice applies if you are taking cyclophosphamide, prescribed to damp down the immune response after organ transplant and increase the chances of the transplant taking. *Astragalus* invigorates the immune system and can, therefore, counteract cyclophosphamide's effects.

The recommended dose of *Astragalus* is 100–150 milligrams daily.

Eating stress-beating foods

Besides antioxidant-rich vegetables and fruit, which do so much to protect and strengthen the immune system, other foods can provide a major resource against the toxic effects of stress, particularly carbohydrates and protein, and those rich in certain minerals.

You may not feel like eating when stress is acute, but most people suffer the effects of stress as part of the everyday pattern of their lives. At such times, stress-beating foods come into their own.

However, when your stomach is in knots and the tension intense, drink lots of extra water and add freshly squeezed and comfortingly delicious fruit and vegetable juices too. In other words, treat yourself to a little extra pleasure with juice from fruits such as raspberry, strawberry, mango, and blueberry, as well as your usual apple, celery, and carrot.

Carbohydrates

If you crave sweet or starchy foods, you probably become irritable and edgy when deprived of them, so the low-G.I. (slow-sugar-release) carbohydrates you eat while detoxing should appeal to you. (refer to Chapter 5, which explains the G.I. rating system.) You get plenty of low-G.I. foods on your detox regimen! They help to guard against mood swings and prevent cravings, thereby boosting your mood and reducing the stress you are under.

It's also worth noting that carbohydrates affect men and women differently. If you are a man, you are more likely to feel calm after eating low-G.I. foods, whereas a woman may feel both calm *and* drowsy.

Young males often do better with a breakfast based on wholegrain cereal or bread, because it helps to combat anxiety and tension during the early part of the day. Whether you're male or female, if you are over 40, you're better off avoiding a high carbohydrate lunch when you need to be mentally alert and able to concentrate during the afternoon.

Protein

Stress increases your need for protein, partly because your body has to manufacture more hormones, enzymes, and other chemicals at an increased rate because of your 'high alert', detoxifying state. Make sure that you are getting your full protein quota when going through traumatic times. Concentrating on typical detox foods such as fresh fruit and veg and obtaining your necessary amino acids from plant protein is kinder to your digestive and excretory organs, and should leave you feeling more balanced, sooner, than a diet high in red meat.

Because of the beneficial effects the amino acid tyrosine has on stressed people, you need to include foods rich in this naturally occurring mood chemical during (and after) detox. Your body makes tyrosine from the essential amino phenylalanine, which is present in most protein food. Especially rich sources include almonds, lima beans, walnuts, and chickpeas.

The amino acid tryptophan increases the level in the brain of the mood booster chemical serotonin, and brings a natural sense of calm and improved ability to cope if you eat it consistently when stressed. Tryptophan also combats depression and mood swings, dulls the sensation of pain, and encourages deep, restful sleep. Foods rich in tryptophan include lamb, liver, roast beef, trout, and pumpkin seeds. Pumpkin seeds are of particular relevance during detox, because they supply antioxidant vitamins and minerals, and because their oil is rich in omega-6 oils (both of which strengthen the beleaguered immune system at times of high stress). Other useful tryptophan sources include chicken breast, cod, roasted peanuts and sesame seeds, soya products, cottage cheese, Brazil nuts, and skimmed milk.

Calcium

Calcium directly offsets the toxic effects of stress and helps to induce inner feelings of tranquillity and calmness. Besides milk and milk products such as cheese and yoghurt, foods rich in calcium include sardines, salmon, soya beans, walnuts, and peanuts. Include these foods in your meals as you approach the end of your detox.

Obviously, you are not smoking during your detox! But it's worth mentioning that smokers (and ex-smokers) need extra calcium, as do women from around the age of 30 onwards, to offset the risks of osteoporosis (the bone-thinning disease) after the menopause.

Magnesium

Magnesium is known as the anti-stress mineral because it is such an effective buffer of stress-induced toxins. It improves nerve and muscle function and also helps in the conversion of blood glucose into energy, always in heavy demand when you're detoxing, and generally, under stressful conditions. Magnesium can also help boost your mood, which can be helpful during detox and at other times.

You need extra magnesium if your alcohol intake has been high, and if you take any form of synthetic oestrogen, for example the contraceptive pill.

Magnesium-rich foods include: wholegrain cereals; corn on the cob; maize flour; nuts (especially almonds); seeds; green vegetables such as spinach, calabrese, broccoli, and parsley; citrus fruit; apples; and figs.

Chapter 9

Embracing Relaxation

- -

- -

*I*f you ever claimed that you have no time for 20 – 30 minutes of dedicated exercise each day, you're even less likely to believe that you have time for complete relaxation. However, relaxation in some form is essential to life – not only for combating stress-generated toxins, but also because prolonged stress eventually causes both physical and mental health problems. Stress has never been more prevalent in our society; official figures released in March 2004 showed a record figure of nearly one million Britons claiming Incapacity Benefit for mental and behavioural disorders, precipitated by stress. An unknown number, doubtless much higher, are off work or otherwise incapacitated due to the physical effects of stress.

Stress aggravates your toxin overload by generating free radicals, which are harmful, overactive oxygen fragments in the tissues and organs. Free radicalsattack and weaken your immune defence system, making it more difficult for your body to cope with toxins it takes in daily due to toxic habits and lifestyle.

You need to learn to relax, in order to overcome stress's negative effects, and this chapter tells you how to do just that. You also discover how certain types of exercise can beat stress and tension, and improve your detox results and vigour.

Rationalising Relaxation

Many factors you may not suspect of adding to your stress do exactly that. Examples include inner tension arising from challenging situations (refer to Chapter 8), lack of exercise (because your wound-up emotions have no healthy outlet), and many of the less-than-healthy foods and drinks you may have been taking regularly such as high intakes of alcohol, caffeine-heavy coffee, tea and cola drinks, and saturated fat are examples. Others include apparently harmless snacks and ready-prepared meals high in hidden fats and refined sugar and flour, not to mention E-number food additives (refer to Chapter 6) used to make and keep food more attractive.

The above factors prevent you from relaxing fully, and benefiting your body and mind when 'at rest'. Examples of their effects include tension headaches and insomnia, anxiety and depression, increased susceptibility to minor ailments and infections, and life-threatening diseases such as cancer, heart disease, and many other conditions including premature ageing.

Not being relaxed increases the risks of the above unpleasant disorders, and detracts from your efforts to detox because continued stress (not relaxing) piles back the toxins into your body just as your excretory organs are trying to drive them out. The result is that you feel exhausted, miserable, and generally off-colour. Relaxation combats the injurious effects of stress, and aids the detox process throughout.

Many people who seriously need to practise relaxation put up a certain amount of resistance when their doctor suggests the idea. Men are less inclined than women to take up the suggestion and both sexes claim not only that they have no time to relax in, but also that they are unable to relax if they do try. However, you are likely to be one of the vast majority of people who *can* learn to switch off. As with every form of self-therapy, some of us are better at it than others, but the tool is one you need if you want to combat the effects of toxins in your body and beat the disorders they bring about. Further benefits include improved sleep, better concentration, and enhanced mental performance.

Making Your Muscles Relax

The gateway to relaxing 'all over' – physically and mentally – is to relax all the main muscles of the body. You cannot quieten an over-stressed mind and body, if you are hunched up, muscles clenched, and breathing in short, rapid bursts as though you'd run a mile.

All this clenching and rapid respiration is not the cause of your stress, but the result. All the same, your muscles are an obvious starting point because you have control of them (as opposed to, say, your adrenal glands, which pump out the high stress hormone, cortisol).

Muscular relaxation also makes you *feel* much better fairly quickly. Breathing is also important, and a minute spent taking slow, deep breaths at the beginning of a relaxation session, sets the pace for overall tension-beating success.

The exercises in the following sections should remind you what muscular tension feels like and how it contrasts with its opposite, muscular relaxation. By serially contracting and relaxing muscle groups throughout your body, starting with your feet and legs and working upwards, you find out which of your muscles need special attention. Doing the exercises also distracts your mind from negative repetitive thoughts and worries and, by soothing the body, help to bring mental tranquillity and peace.

Wear loose comfortable clothing when doing the exercises – pyjamas or a tracksuit are ideal.

Pick a time when you can be left quietly alone for 20–30 minutes and switch off any extraneous noises such as the radio and the television. When you are adept at relaxation you may choose to play peaceful, gentle music as a relaxation aid.

The basic routine is the same for all the muscle groups.Start by lying on a comfortable rug on the floor. Then, for each muscle group I mention below, do as follows:

1. **Tense and hold for 15–20 seconds**.

   Note how this feels.

2. **Say 'relax' to yourself and let the tension go.**

   Focus on the difference in feeling between the two states.

3. **Enjoy the contrast between your relaxed and tensed muscles for 20–30 seconds.**

4. **Repeat once or twice more, until the muscles you are working on feel generally less taut and strung-out. Then move on to another group.**

Focus on the muscle groups in the same order as the following subsections.

Legs and feet

Work on each side in turn.

> ✔ **Toes and feet:** Curl your toes by trying to bring the tips down to the ball of your foot – not hard enough to give you cramp, but hard enough to feel the pull. Then uncurl and move on.

✔ **Lower legs:** Bend your toes and feet downwards at the ankle and squeeze the muscles you can feel pulling, tightening the calf muscles; next, flex your ankles to point your toes and feet towards your face, tightening the muscle groups at the front and side of your calves. Relax.

✔ **Thighs:** Straighten and stiffen your legs, and lift your feet upwards off the floor, to tense the muscles at the front of your thighs, then bend slightly at your knees to flex the muscles on the backs of your thighs. Then relax.

Trunk

The whole exercise consists of relaxing each muscle group in turn. While you're still down on the floor on your rug, try the following:

✔ **Stomach:** Pull in your stomach and then push it out.

✔ **Buttocks:** Squeeze and relax.

✔ **Back:** Arch and relax.

✔ **Chest:** Take a deep breath and hold it, then let it go and relax.

Arms and hands

While you are lying on the ground, try each of the following in turn:

✔ **Hands and forearms:** Lift your arms in the air above you; make a tight fist, and bend your forearms downwards at the elbows. Relax.

✔ **Biceps (fronts of upper arms):** Make a 'muscle' on both your arms, the 'strongman' pose you did to impress your friends when you were ten. You'll see and feel the biceps bulging like an egg. Hold, then relax and lower your arms.

✔ **Triceps (backs of upper arms):** Stretch your arms straight up in the air again, and tense the backs of your upper arms. Lower your arms to the floor again, and relax.

Upper body

While you're still on the floor on the mat, try the following:

✔ **Shoulders:** Shrug your shoulders to get them as close to your ears as possible and roll them backwards and forwards. Bring them back to your ears and let them sag.

Taking a minute to relax

Your boss just made another impossible demand. Your child wreaked havoc in the kitchen just making a snack! You're stuck in traffic with no movement in sight. You are completely stressed out, ready to explode. Before you do damage to yourself or others, take just a moment to calm down, thereby saving your sanity and your health.

Firstly take two to three very slow, very deep breaths. The slow breathing slows your heart rate and quietens some of your tense systems. Then sit down and utilise just a fraction of your relaxation routine. Make a tight fist with your left hand, for example, squeeze for 2 to 3 seconds and feel the tightness in your hand, wrist and forearms. Then, gently relax. As you perform the actions, say, 'Tennnnse . . . relaaaaax' in a gentle, drawn-out way.

Next, contract your biceps (the muscle group on the front of your upper arm) and again, still breathing slowly and deeply, repeat the words, 'Tennnnse . . . relaaaaax'. Feel the tightness in your upper arm, followed by the delightful, 'letting go' sensation of relaxation. Then straighten your arm at the elbow and squeeze all the muscles as hard as you can without hurting yourself, saying again, 'Tennnnse . . . relaaaaax'.

It's a good idea to prepare this exercise in advance so that you are ready when high stress strikes. Rehearse it straight after a normal relaxation session: picture something that normally stresses you, such as being tailgated while driving, or trying to guess your way through an automated telephone answer system, and picture the stressful situation becoming squeezed into the tightness of your whole arm, following each squeeze with completely loose, floppy, limp relaxation. The passing of the tension out of each muscle group symbolises – in fact is – the sluicing out of your anger, fear, frustration, or other negative feelings, together with the tissue toxins they induce.

If you cannot get away from the stressful situation or person, you can make do with a single clenched fist. Clench it as tightly as you can, for one minute. Drive all your negative emotions and tension down into the iron-hard muscles, hold them there for 15 to 20 seconds, then release them, letting your stress trickle away as you relax. Repeat 'Tennnnse . . . relaaaaax' under your breath, or just say them in your mind.

✔ **Neck:** Raise your body from the floor slightly, so you're propped up on your forearms. Roll your head right around in a circle, up, to your right, downwards, up to your left, and finally upwards to the ceiling.

✔ **Jaw:** Clench your jaws, then let go.

✔ **Forehead:** Frown hard, then raise your eyebrows. Relax.

✔ **Lips:** Press your lips together, then relax.

✔ **Tongue:** Stick out your tongue, then put it in and press it against the roof of your mouth. Relax.

Total body relaxation

Still lying on the mat, check each of the previous muscle groups in turn, and repeat the tensing/letting go routine for any group in which you still notice any tension.

1. **Tell yourself that you feel warm, comfortable, and relaxed all over.**

2. **Imagine that you are floating gently down a perfumed stream, strewn with rose petals.**

3. **Count down slowly from ten to one, enjoying the dappled sunlight, the shade, the birds, and the flowers.**

   You are feeling more and more deeply relaxed as you approach a small, secret pool where you come gently to rest, perfectly relaxed and at peace.

4. **Enjoy your time in the secret pool.**

5. **Count up slowly from one to ten when you wish to come out of this state.**

   Say to yourself: 'To wake up, I am going to count from 1 to 10. By the time I reach ten, I shall be wide awake and refreshed. 1 . . . 2 . . . 3 . . . 4 . . . 5 . . . I am waking up . . . 6 . . . 7 . . . 8 . . . I am stretching and opening my eyes . . . 9 . . . 10 . . . I am fully awake and feeling wonderful.'

Stretching Away Tension with Yoga

Yoga is a life and health improvement system that has been practiced in the East for several thousand years. The best known yoga in Britain is Indian in origin, and its life-enhancing benefits are felt (when practiced regularly) in: reduced tension levels; improved ability to deal with stress and negative emotions; many health improvements such as certain types of high blood pressure; improvements in nervous complaints such as palpitation and poor sleep; and greater resources of vitality and energy.

Yoga is so popular in the UK that it's almost impossible to find a health club or leisure centre that does not include it in its curriculum. Yoga induces calmness and tranquility, while stretching and working the muscles of the body in certain positions called asanas. Yoga is entirely non-competitive and suitable for almost anyone and at any age.

As you are probably aware, yoga is not only a great stress-beater, it does a great deal more besides. Brief descriptions of the exercises do not give a true impression of the immense relaxation that yoga can bring, and it works on stress at so many levels, becoming an invaluable tool to a healthy, toxin-free lifestyle.

Yoga means 'union' – essentially of individual consciousness (known as jivatman) and the universal consciousness (paramatman). Yoga also brings harmony and balance to the body, mind and spirit. Like deep relaxation, yoga creates an altered state of awareness *and* instructs and shows its followers how the altered state can be achieved.

The *asanas,* or 'steady poses', are the basis of yoga. If you practise the poses regularly, you enhance the flexibility and proper function of your spine, which in turn maximises the delivery of oxygen and nutrients to the spinal chord, brain, and those nerves that travel from the brain and spinal chord to your upper body areas.

Many of the asanas also strengthen and harmonise the body's stress control systems, including the hypothalamus and pituitary gland in the brain, and other endocrine glands, including the adrenals, in the body. These systems all go into overdrive when you're under strain, or having to deal with uncontrollable stress.

Yoga has become evermore widely accepted since the 1960s, and in most leisure centres, evening-class programmes, and fitness groups in Britain counts among the most highly-subscribed activities. Contact a centre to find a class near you or pick up an instructional book or video – preferably one of the many *For Dummies* books (www.dummies.com) DVDs on the subject.

Thinking (Or Not Thinking) Your Way to Relaxation through Meditation

Once you grasp the need for and feel positive about regular relaxation, it's but a small step to consideration of meditation as a regular practise. Meditation is a resource for calming the mind and emotions. Many people shy away from it because they do not know anything about it, but the health benefits are proven in many hundreds of clinical studies and meditation is simple to do. The description below outlines a simple meditation method.

The good thing about meditation is that it conveys benefits from the day you start practising it, and its effects are cumulative.

Ultimately, when you've practised meditation for a long time, the change in consciousness can provide a sense of blissful tranquillity, freeing you to cope with highly adverse circumstances without becoming depressed, anxious or stressed.

To put into practice a simple meditation session, set aside 30 minutes of your day when you can be alone and can unplug the telephone and maybe leave a note on your front door saying that you do not wish to be disturbed.

Have a shower or bath if you have time, and put on simple and undemanding clothes to make you feel relaxed and at ease. Then follow these steps:

1. **Sit down on a floor cushion or on a straight-backed chair, in a dimly lit room with all possible noise quelled.**

   You can light a candle, if you wish, and warm a soothing aromatherapy oil of your choice in an aromatherapy oil heater.

2. **Sit comfortably and breathe deeply and slowly.**

   Relax each muscle group in turn as described in the first section of this chapter.

   Feel and hear the breath slowly entering your body, hold it for a few seconds and exhale slowly.

3. **Concentrate only on your breathing.**

   Focus on how your chest and lungs feel as you breathe. Just concentrate on the *in* breath, the *holding* of the breath, and the *exhaling*. If other thoughts arise, acknowledge them and let them go. The harder you try to banish them, the longer they stick around.

   Notice how calm and free you feel, and how extraneous thoughts slowly start to disappear.

4. **Hold this state for as long as you can.**

   You'll know when you have had enough. Aim for 10 minutes at first and gradually increase to 20 minutes daily. How long you're able to meditate will increase as you persist with your practice.

When you practise meditation, you remain fully conscious and aware of your surroundings, but you become increasingly free of the thoughts that persistently present themselves throughout your normal waking hours.

By banishing familiar mental stresses and strains you achieve a brain function at which your mind is most effective. Problems and minor irritations appear in proportion and you come to realise that trivial troubles truly are of no importance and that even larger ones eventually pass.

In fact, it has been suggested that through the practise of meditation you can develop your innate sixth sense, such as clairvoyance.

Getting High-Quality Sleep

Quality sleep, from which you awake feeling refreshed and invigorated, is essential to physical and mental health, but is also a prime antidote to stress-induced toxins. The body really does rejuvenate during sleep.

Not getting enough sleep or enough quality sleep is a source of both mental and physical stress. You can no doubt identify with the 'toxic' feeling that comes with staying up all night or crossing several time zones and feeling jet-lagged.

The following subsections address the likely causes of disturbed sleep and offer tips on how to cope with each.

Suffering from sleep apnoea

Sleep apnoea is a major cause of disturbed sleep, but one from which you may not be aware you're suffering. Sleep apnoea has many possible causes – it can be prompted by your being overweight, being over a certain age, or drinking a lot of alcohol before retiring, among other reasons. The way it works is that the muscles of the neck and throat relax so much that the upper airway is obstructed as you snooze. Your sleep is interrupted after short intervals throughout the night because of a lack of oxygen getting to your brain, due to the throat obstruction, and this partly wakes you.

Sufferers typically give a jump and a choking sort of snort before waking, turning over, dropping off to sleep, waking, turning over, dropping off to sleep, over and over throughout the night.

A sleep-wake-sleep cycle destroys the benefit of deep quality rest and the repeated drops in blood oxygen levels, which results from the partial throat obstruction, has been convincingly linked to an increased risk of a heart attack.

If you think that you may suffer from sleep apnoea, see your doctor. He or she may advise you to lose weight, stop smoking, cut back on alcohol, and possibly use a specially-designed throat spray, which helps to combat the problem. Other possibilities include an assessment at a sleep laboratory to study your sleep patterns and suggest other treatments for your sleep apnoea as required.

Snoring the night away

If your snoring does not wake you, you may well be woken several times every night by your frustrated and wakeful partner. Alternatively, your sleeping partner may be the snorer, and *you* may suffer disturbed sleep nightly.

Various treatments are available from mail order companies and pharmacists, including throat sprays: Sleep Wizard, a lightweight jaw support that keeps your lower jaw forward while you're asleep, combating both snoring and sleep apnoea (see www.sleepwizard. com); and Sleep Pro (see www.sleeppro.com), which is a device you insert in your mouth before switching off for the night. The device holds your lower jaw forward, and minimises both snoring and sleep apnoea.

If nothing eases the snoring, your GP may refer you to an ear, nose, and throat surgeon, who may discuss the possibility of corrective surgery. You can also help yourself by losing excess weight, drinking less alcohol, and sleeping on your side.

To ensure that you sleep on your side, sew a tennis ball into the back of your pyjamas or nightdress. Rolling onto the ball should rouse you sufficiently to get you off your back and onto your side again.

Blaming addictive substances

I mention heavy drinking as a cause for sleep disturbances in both preceding subsections. It can also ruin your night's rest by giving rise to bad dreams, numerous trips to the bathroom, and both hangover and alcohol withdrawal symptoms. You may think that passing lots of urine, nausea and vomiting, thumping headaches, diarrhoea, sweating, and stomach pains are an acceptable price to pay for an evening's binge drinking but, if you're serious about your detox, stop pursuing such 'pleasure'. In addition to the risky blood pressure rise and organ damage it causes, very heavy drinking also deprives you of vital relaxation and increases the toxic harm that your drinking and other stress factors create.

Dependence on sedative drugs such as temazepam and zopiclone can also interfere with healthy sleep, and although you are likely to experience sleep disturbance while coming off them, make sure that you review your night-time medication with your doctor without delay.

Tossing and turning with worry, anxiety, and depression

Nearly everyone worries at some time. You don't accomplish anything by worrying about it, and you are no doubt aware that few of the things people worry about ever materialise (at least not in the dire form that can take over your imagination). Nevertheless, it can be extremely difficult to get rid of worry once it sets in.

I recommend an excellent book on the subject, which can help you see worry in a new light, and hopefully get a handle on your own: *The Easy Way To Stop Worrying,* by Alan Carr (Arcturus Foulsham).

Anxiety differs from worry in that (among other ways) an underlying psychological cause always exists for the symptoms in addition to whatever you are ostensibly fretting about. Anxiety gets more out of hand than 'simple' worry, and affects many areas of your health and life. Sound sleep is one of the most important of these areas.

If you suffer from uncontrollable anxiety, panic attacks, phobias, or other anxiety-related disorders, see your GP, if you haven't already done so, for advice and treatment.

Anxiety is often a feature of depression, and in this case, your sleep is likely to be poor in quality and diminished in time – partly because you find it hard to get to sleep (you're tossing and turning instead) and equally hard to remain asleep. Your sleep is also likely to be broken by dreams and to leave you feeling like a wrung-out dishrag in the morning.

Endogenous depression – the kind that arises for no apparent cause – also causes disturbed sleep. You fall asleep relatively quickly but are prey to early-morning waking. You may wake at 3 o'clock or 4 o'clock in the morning after only four or five hours' sleep, and be unable to drop off again – tossing and turning fretfully for the rest of the night until the alarm clock rings.

If you believe you are depressed, see your doctor for advice and treatment without delay.

Relieving bad sleep experiences

You may lie awake night after night unable to sleep (although desperately tired) because all attempts to treat your insomnia have failed. Or, perhaps, you have been prescribed sleeping drugs for a short time with a view to rebalancing your sleeping habits, and you are no better off now they have been withdrawn. Unsurprisingly, you are now convinced that your sick sleeping habit is incurable and that you simply have to put up with the lack of sleep.

This situation is very rarely, if ever, the case. Firstly, few insomniacs fail to benefit from a referral to a sleep laboratory where doctors and other sleep specialists keep track of your sleep (or lack of it) overnight using electronic monitoring equipment. Suggestions and treatment are forthcoming once the pattern and cause of your poor sleep are fully explored.

You can also try psychological treatments, the best-known of which is hypnotherapy. If the therapist is able to plant a post-hypnotic suggestion in your subconscious mind that, after a little ritual such as blowing your nose, sipping water, and turning off your bedside light, you will go to, and stay, beneficially asleep, then you are highly likely to do exactly that. (Check *Hypnotherapy For Dummies,* by Michael Bryant and Peter Mabbutt (Wiley) for more on hypnotherapy.)

Tranquil music of dolphin and whale calls, a waterfall, gentle rain, and other desirable sounds are widely available on tape and CD and can work alone or in conjunction with other self-help advice. Look for them on the Internet, or enquire about them in your local health food shop, or a shop specialising in fair-trade goods and ethnic health and relaxation products.

Part IV
Planning Your Detox

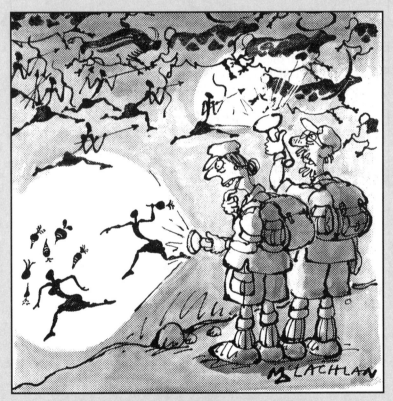

"I think we've just discovered the very first attempt to persuade man to detox."

In this part . . .

*I*t is easy to plan your own detox specifically suited to your personal requirements and here I show you how. I also provide a choice of plans of different length for you to consider. I give you advice on each choice, taking into account your detox experience (or lack of it), and the time you have available.

In Chapter 11 I describe herbal and nutritional supplements that can help the detox process, and explain when and how to use them. I give advice on dosage, and details of supplements that can generally be found with ease through your health food store, pharmacy, or online.

Chapter 12 covers essential information on maintaining detox for life. By the time you finish your first detox, you will surely wish to continue receiving the benefits of your efforts on a daily basis thereafter. Here I tell you how!

Chapter 10

DIY Detox

*I*n this chapter, I tell you how to customise your detox so that it suits your personal needs. I show you how to decide on such things as which protein foods to select (fish, poultry, or vegetarian), how intensive (or gentle) you want your detox to be, and how long it should last.

Next, you find out about about forward planning, a most important stage which radically decreases the chances of your quitting before the detox programme is over. Follow the tips on mental and physical preparation, and the five-day count-down to 'Detox day one', and you will find the transition from toxic lifestyle to detox cleansing and renewal simpler than you can have imagined.

Finally, you read about three different detox plans – weekend, 7-day and 14-day programmes. Each of these includes tips on exercise, relaxation, meal choices, water intake, and the use of supplementary cleansing and revitalising aids such as aromatherapy essences, massage, and fresh fruit and vegetable juices.

Planning Your Own Detox Programme

Hopefully, you're looking forward to planning your detox programme. You need to decide on how long you want your detox to last, what areas to concentrate on, how much exercise and/or rest you intend to take, and which kind of protein you're going to eat.

Measuring the length

How long you decide to detox for depends upon the time you have available, whether you have detoxed before, and any special needs that arise in connection with your lifestyle. Here are points you may like to consider when selecting your detox length.

- The **24-hour detox:** likely to suit you if you have detoxed before – perhaps you detox regularly (for instance, twice yearly). You may need to 'top up' the cleansing and balancing process between detoxes, or combat the effects of an eating or drinking splurge (and yes, detoxers **do** fall by the wayside at times). Regular detoxing aids your health and immune defence, but it does not transform you into a neurotic health freak – or a saint! A suitable regimen for a single day detox would be Day One of any of the three programmes that I provide at the end of this chapter.

- The **weekend detox:** this may be right for you as a first-time detoxer and if you don't have the opportunity to spend a whole week on a detox plan. It's a frequent choice of regular detoxers.

- The **7-day detox:** this is probably your best choice if you're completely new to the detox process. You need a day or two to acclimatise yourself to the cleansing phase and if you experience mild side effects such as headaches, a bad taste in your mouth, or tiredness, you need time to get used to what is happening in your body, and remind yourself of the massive benefits in store. Detoxing calmly and thoughtfully will help you to benefit from the suggested periods of relaxation and rest (see Planning your 7-day detox later in this chapter). You should also have increased vitality and feel 'born again' as you complete the balancing and reinvigorating stage.

- **The 14-day detox:** this is probably best suited to you if you are an old hand at detoxing, and have experience of sticking to shorter detoxes satisfactorily. For example, you may choose to detox for a fortnight rather than your usual week, if your vitality and energy levels have been especially low in recent months, or you have been subjected to an unusual degree of exposure to everyday toxins such as tobacco smoke, alcohol and processed foods.

Choosing where to concentrate

You can get an idea of how toxic your diet and lifestyle is now by using the information from Part III of this book. You must then decide on which aspect(s) of cleansing you most need to concentrate on. To help you make up your mind, the following subsections assist you in discovering which of your eliminatory organs are working overtime on your behalf.

Groaning gut?

If you're a food junkie, or eat masses of red meat, your bowel may be clogged with putrifying waste. (I am not going to define 'masses of red meat' – it depends upon your individual physique, exercise output and requirements, but most nutritionists agree that 75–100g (3–4 oz) daily suffices for the average person.)

A bowel stuffed with waste works sluggishly at best and can give rise to fatigue, a pasty complexion, excess weight that just doesn't go however hard you try, a bad taste in the mouth, and bad breath.

You need sufficient energy to do a little brisk walking, yoga or similar exercise to help your bowel to work regularly again. See below for your best choice of detox foods (for supplements, see Chapter 11).

Loopy lungs?

If you're a smoker, detox should prove a real treat. Your breathing becomes easier and the circulation to your muscles and heart improves. (Refer to Chapter 3.)

To help bring these goodies about, leave time for yoga and gentle exercise (refer to Chapter 9) to improve your breathing and make especially sure to eat fruit and vegetables rich in beta-carotene (pro-vitamin A), plus other cancer-fighting oxidants. (Refer to Chapter 5, which talks about good detox foods.)

Think, too, in terms of regular snacks – sunflower seeds to help beat nicotine cravings, and other low-G.I. (low glycaemic index) carbohydrates to reduce irritability and nervous tension. (Refer to Chapter 5, which has a G.I. table you can consult.)

Languishing liver?

You'll know well enough whether your liver needs first consideration in your detox plan. Firstly, you'll be aware that you have exceeded the recommended intake of 14 units/week (for a woman), or 21 units (for a man) – a unit is a half pint of beer or lager, 125 millilitre standard strength wine, that is, 12% abv, a single pub measure of spirits or a pub schooner of fortified wine such as sherry or vermouth.

Secondly, you'll be aware of having frequent hangovers, feeling nauseous, out-of-sorts and possibly depressed, and may have fleeting pains in the upper right part of your abdomen, which your GP assures you is not due to an inflamed gall bladder.

Alcohol misuse, which produces liver tenderness, eventually reveals itself in blood tests.

Plan to take gentle exercise, eat a moderate amount of protein foods and as little fat as possible. You'll also benefit from relaxation and rest to help you recover from your (final?) hangover, and calm your nerves should alcohol cravings set in.

Crotchety kidneys?

Are you chronically dehydrated? Probably you are, if you drink fewer than 5–6 glasses of water (250 millilitres or 10 fluid ounces) daily, and fill yourself up with caffeine-rich cola, and mugs of coffee and tea.

Long-standing water shortage not only compromises your kidneys' ability to manufacture urine and filter out toxins, it also prevents your other systems and organs from working as they should.

Constipation, a muddy complexion, skin rashes, dry mouth and tongue, bad taste in the mouth and awful breath, are all signs of kidney neglect.

You won't be drinking caffeine-rich beverages or alcohol (another dehydrator) while detoxing, so drink a glass of water (see above) 5–6 times day to help your kidneys work at full capacity.

Also, think in terms of moderate exercise to crank up your circulation – in this way your kidneys receive lots of oxygen-rich blood, and form plenty of urine to eliminate many water-soluble toxins.

Scowling skin?

Your skin is your largest (although not your most obvious) excretory organ, and it's easily taken for granted. You're probably aware of the dangers of the sun's UV rays, and, if you burn easily, you should wear a sunscreen in strong sunlight.

But less sunny days can also produce enough UV radiation to generate free radicals. These hyperactive oxygen fragments act as toxins in your skin, impairing its toxin-eliminating actions and giving rise to premature age changes, puffiness, lines, and wrinkles. When your skin is out of condition, it works less efficiently so that fewer toxins are expelled in your sweat, adding to your toxin overload.

If you've damaged your skin by not providing it with nutrients, or it has become dehydrated, or you have not been using sun screens and moisturisers, choose a detox scheme with moderate exercise (your skin needs freshly oxygenated blood pumping round its cells and extracting toxic waste). You also need masses of antioxidants (present in pulses, nuts, grains, and legumes as well as fresh fruit and vegetables), restful sleep, and some skin-nourishing treats, in addition to ample water.

Stress excess?

You know whether you're over-stressed – you feel exhausted all the time, are tense, anxious, possibly depressed, and maybe sleep badly (refer back to Chapter 8 for an explanation of the causes and symptoms of stress).

The sort of detox programme most suited to your needs provides ample rest, allowing you time to practise relaxation techniques (several are explained in Chapter 9).

Your best detox foods are rich both in antioxidants (so lots of fresh fruit and vegetables), and in tryptophan. The brain converts this amino acid into the tension-beating nerve messenger serotonin. Foods rich in tryptophan include lamb, liver, turkey, chicken breast, shrimps, cod, trout, soya products, cottage cheese and skimmed milk, brazil nuts, and pumpkin and sesame seeds. Other benefits of tryptophan-rich detox foods include a brighter mood, fewer mood swings, more refreshing sleep, and a higher pain threshold. This means that you experience less discomfort than usual from such long-standing painful conditions as backache, muscular aches and pains, and arthritis.

 Choose a moderately active detox scheme (unless physical exhaustion is part of your problem) because active exercise provides an outlet for pent-up emotional tension. Aerobic exercise can also lead to the release of *endorphins* – morphine-related brain chemicals that lift the mood and can produce euphoria.

Taking it easy (or not)

You know from your lifestyle, and any weight problems you may have, as well as your overall health and vitality, whether you're crying out, body and soul, for masses of lovely rest or whether exerting yourself would provide more benefit (even though you may not 'feel like it').

Exercise can be very beneficial during a detox, but you *must* go easy at first to avoid overtaxing your strength. If you are accustomed to high blood sugar levels, are a heavy drinker, or are suffering from exhaustion, take only light exercise such as simple stretches and gentle walking.

Lots of rest is also essential, and you can enjoy 'doing nothing' for a few hours every day with a clear conscience, because resting your body (and mind) are essential to the detox process!

All your excretory organs depend upon blood to bring them nutrients and oxygen, as well as the toxins which they remove. So, keeping your circulatory system running smoothly is essential. And exercise, whether mild or strenuous, gets your blood pumping.

The cleansing and rejuvenating processes of detox are bound to make you more tired than usual, at least for the first day or so. You may be eating more healthily, and taking in more low G.I. (low glycaemic index) foods, but your body – especially your gut and liver – needs time to adjust to the changes.

Always allow your own body and energy levels to dictate what is best for *you*. Someone of the same age and sex who is equally used to sugary junk foods, lots of alcohol, and high stress levels may react quite differently when following a similar detox plan to the way you do.

Some gentle yoga practice (refer to Chapter 9) should benefit you whichever form of detox you choose.

Picking your protein

You may have already selected the sort of protein foods you're going to eat during your detox. Excellent choices are vegetarian dishes combining grains, pulses and nuts to provide the full complement of essential amino acids (protein building blocks). Fish and the lean meat of poultry and fowl can also be eaten towards the end of detox, when you are reintroducing the sort of healthy foods you can eat after detox is over.

The latter may, of course, include red meat, but this is excluded from detox plans because of its hidden saturated fat content, the artificial farming toxins it can contain (such as antibiotics and growth enhancers) and the relatively heavy task it imposes on your digestive organs compared with lighter protein sources. After all, you are trying to encourage your intestine to *throw off* accumulated debris and toxic waste, much of which is believed to come from red meat (in meat eaters) in the first place.

This may be stating the obvious, but taste – your personal likes and dislikes – is extremely important. If you loathe, or are allergic, to fish (for example) you avoid it, however attracted you are by its health benefits. Detox is demanding, but *not* a punishment for lifestyle or dietary 'sins' of the past! Choose the foods you enjoy – your mood as you eat affects digestion and possibly how your body uses various nutrients as well.

Having said this, I urge you to try foods you may not have eaten before (lentils and pomegranates, for instance), and give others you disliked as a child a second chance. Many people think that they hate porridge, but its popularity with slimming celebrities has recently increased its profile as a popular breakfast choice. Even those who refuse to eat vegetables can be coaxed into sampling a few garden peas, baby carrots, or cherry tomatoes, and end up liking them.

Catching on to fish

Fish is an excellent choice for, well, fish lovers, as well as those who wish to optimise the health of their brain, heart, and circulation or suffer from high blood pressure, high cholesterol, heart disease, or poor circulation generally.

Choose oily fish, such as salmon, tuna, mackerel, sardines, pilchards, kippers, and herring. Rich in omega-3 essential fatty acids, these types not only boost blood flow and brain power, they also relieve the symptoms of osteo- and rheumatoid arthritis, eczema, psoriasis, and possibly other inflammatory conditions. Oily fish is also a great choice if you are diabetic, because it can help decrease your risks of developing heart and blood-vessel disorders to which diabetics are especially prone.

If you are diabetic and planning to detox, make sure that you discuss your plans beforehand with your GP, diabetic nurse, or other health professional.

Salmon is delicious simply microwaved for 2–3 minutes, covered, on medium power and with a little water. Most oily fish can be dry-fried, fried in a hot pan without any oil, to avoid adding fat and energy calories. This seals in the juices and, because you apply heat to both sides and the temperature is high, the interior of the protein food cooks, too.

Plucking fowl

Most people like at least one variety of fowl or poultry. Chicken and turkey – excellent sources of the amino acid tryptophan which helps regulate moods – and other land fowl such as pigeon, pheasant, snipe, and grouse have fairly 'dry' meat that provides good, tasty protein (even without the skin!).

The flesh of water birds such as duck and goose is notoriously greasy. Avoid it while detoxing and eat it sparingly at other times!

Here's a 'naughty' tip that you can indulge in, once in a while. After virtuously removing your poultry's skin, help yourself to the tail bit, known as the parson's nose – utterly delectable, juicy, and contains just enough fat to compensate for the 'treat' you otherwise miss.

Choose poultry for your protein if you need meat (as opposed to oily fish or vegetables) to suit a delicate digestion, and/or suffer from depression, longstanding anxiety and stress, chronic pain or poor quality sleep. While a single meal makes no apparent difference, many people who suffer mood disorders find that eating poultry regularly brings relief.

Sorting through beans and pulses

Beans and pulses may not have the cachet of, say, Parma ham or truffles, but many people who experiment with them find them unexpectedly delicious. It's also a fact that practically everyone on earth who tries baked beans loves them, and they are just haricot beans, one of the major pulses, tinned and served in sauce. (For a healthy, detox version, try out the recipe in Chapter 13.)

Legumes, that is, beans, lentils, and peas, are also excellent food for would-be slimmers during detox, although the opposite may seem to be the case if you're unfamiliar with low G.I. dieting. Their disadvantage is that they make some people (although by no means all) windy. But they're fibre and nutrient-rich, filling, and release sugars steadily into the bloodstream without over-boosting your blood glucose level. They're also extremely adaptable, taking well to simple dressings such as soy sauce, lemon juice, and herbs (for example).

Preparing for Take-Off

If you're itching to get going – maybe even thinking: 'Why can't I just *start,* instead of wasting time with preparation?,' then it's worth knowing that making small lifestyle and dietary changes beforehand helps your detox run more smoothly.

Even the gentlest detox makes physical and mental demands upon you, and you need to damp down the therapeutic, but occasionally somewhat brisk, shock to the system detox can cause. Plunging without warning into detox is like waking up, groggy after a deep sleep and diving headfirst into an icy pool. A bracing wake-up call, certainly – but kinder, less traumatic methods are advisable.

The cleansing stage, in particular, (Chapter 4 explains the three stages of detox – cleansing, balancing, and fortifying) can make you feel washed-out, and give rise to headaches, irritability, bad breath, and a bad taste in the mouth, particularly after a weekend of hearty eating and drinking, for instance, or a period of huge stress. Cutting back for a few days keeps unpleasant symptoms, and cravings, to a minimum.

The tips in the following subsections cover mental/emotional and physical preparation. Some will apply to you, others not. The subsections give advice about the best way to prepare for detoxing if, for example, you are very stressed, smoke, drink heavily, or take lots of medications. Read them through before deciding on the type of detox that best suits your needs.

Being armed with the information in these subsections puts you in a position to plot your detox like a military manoeuvre! The aptness of this analogy soon becomes apparent when you think of the enemy toxins you are going to hound out of your system, aided and abetted by an army of free radical-fighting antioxidants.

Getting ready mentally

Follow these tips for a week, at least, before your detox starts, to prepare your mind and emotions:

Think positive!

Do write down three reasons why you want to detox, wording them as specifically as you can. Some sound choices are

- ✔ Detox is going to give me renewed energy and vigour.
- ✔ Detox is going to improve my health and my enjoyment of life.
- ✔ I want to look and feel years younger, both physically and mentally.

Don't be vague as in 'I want to get rid of toxins.' And don't worry about your decision to detox, fearing that you've insufficient willpower to follow it through.

Concentrate on the benefits!

If you think of detox in terms of what you'll be giving up, you'll probably give in!

It's true you'll be cutting right back on, then eliminating, toxic habits before you start your programme (see the 'Priming your body' section later). This in itself will reduce your cravings during the detox process, but you cannot expect not to miss cigarettes or alcohol – or, indeed, caffeine, refined sugar, or inessential pills and potions – if you're a regular user.

Don't dread your forthcoming detox as something to be endured. *Do* focus upon:

- ✔ Your healthier liver, enjoying its alcohol-free 'gap year', driving out toxins with a will – without any hangover symptoms!

- ✔ Your healthier kidneys, excreting toxins, and lots of retained fluid, making you feel lighter and far less bloated.

- ✔ Your healthier gut, throwing off accumulated waste, and masses of harmful bacteria. You feel lighter, and your bowels remain or become regular.

- ✔ Your healthier, smoke-free lungs, breathing out airborne toxins and taking in extra oxygen, making you feel and smell fresher, cleaner, purified.

- ✔ Your healthier skin, oozing out toxins through cleaner, unclogged pores. Your complexion will clear and, with the extra fluid, your skin will start to look younger.

Make a chart anticipating success!

Once you decide on the length of your detox (the previous section 'Measuring the length' helps you choose), draw up a chart of squares, with the days along the horizontal axis, and the periods of rest and any exercise you mean to do such as yoga and meditation, and any detox meals you plan to eat, along the vertical axis. Visualise yourself ticking them in a cheerful colour, as you progress, stage-by-stage, through your detox plan.

Do decorate the chart with stickers, happy faces, apt quotations, positive thoughts, or whatever you fancy. Stick it up somewhere where you can see it often, and preferably out of sight of anyone (should there *be* anyone) in your household who is cynical or off-putting about your forthcoming achievement.

Don't list possible symptoms, cravings, and so on. Like obsessively studying the leaflet inside a package of prescribed medicine, nothing induces 'side effects' (or symptoms) more thoroughly then being advised to expect them! You'll know soon enough if they occur, and I give you tips on relieving them safely and naturally later in this chapter.

Priming your body

Stress is a major contributor to your toxin overload, and your need to combat it is especially great during a detox programme if you want to ensure that your improved diet and lifestyle changes proceed unhampered. So, the first preparation is to discover and practise relaxation!

Take 20–30 minutes' additional rest during the countdown days and master one of the simple stress-beating measures outlined in Chapter 9. Use as necessary!

If you're a smoker, heavy drinker, or habitual user of inessential medicines, you probably need a month to six weeks in which to cut down, before quitting entirely while detoxing. (Refer to Chapter 7.) Follow the tips there, supplemented by those in the preceding 'Getting ready mentally' section.

You can also picture yourself celebrating a two-fold triumph – completing detox and quitting an antisocial habit which can only harm you and others.

Regarding alcohol, you can, if you wish, look forward to reintroducing some alcohol into your diet after you complete your detox, following the guidelines for safe drinking that I go through in Chapter 7.

Regarding prescription medicines, ask your doctor's advice if you've any doubt about your need to continue taking them. With management targets and the prescriptions budget ever in view (if for no other reason), your GP is unlikely to insist on prescribing drugs unnecessarily.

If you pop over-the-counter medications such as painkillers, anti-inflammatory drugs, laxatives, caffeine-based stimulants, and so on, remember that you're preparing to detoxify your system, not add a welter of unnecessary chemicals. Ease yourself out of the habit, using hints I give later in this chapter for relieving common ailments.

Beginning the countdown

The following subsections outline my suggested 5-day countdown to detox, from day 5 to day 1. Feel free to adapt the routine to suit your personal needs according to your current lifestyle; for instance, whether you drink alcohol, eat a lot of fried food, or take many cups of coffee and tea daily.

The purpose of the countdown is to wean you off foods and drinks you have to eliminate completely during detox. Suddenly ceasing to drink alcohol or strong coffee, refined sugar and junk foods, for example, would be too taxing to you physically and emotionally.

Throughout, you need to eat breakfast, lunch, and an evening meal – with snacks of fresh, raw fruit and vegetables in between if you like.

Day 5

Halve your normal junk food intake – instead of two bars of chocolate – eat just one. If you eat three bags of crisps – eat one and a half!

Halve your cola drinks – for 1 litre of coke, drink 500 millilitres.

Halve your alcohol consumption – three units instead of six, a glass and a half of wine in place of three, two halves of lager instead of two pints. One unit is 125 millilitres 12% abv (standard strength) wine, half a pint of lager or beer, a pub measure of spirits or a pub schooner of sherry or other fortified wine such as vermouth.

Cut out one cup of tea or coffee (if you only drink 1–2 cups a day anyway, you may choose simply to stop).

No more takeaways – avoid food fried in batter, and shallow-fry (using only a little oil) meat, fish, and vegetables instead of deep frying them if applicable.

Eat at least one portion of fresh vegetables or fruit – raw as a salad, with or without a main meal, or as a snack between meals. Dress salad if you wish with a few drops of cider vinegar or a squeeze of fresh lemon or lime juice and some fresh or dried herbs.

Drink at least one glass (250 millilitres, 10 fluid ounces) of water.

Day 4

Halve your junk food intake once again.

Halve your cola drinks.

Halve your alcohol consumption – in the case of wine you can have the same number of glasses, using half wine/half sparkling or still mineral water (otherwise known as a spritzer). Or try low-alcohol wine or beer.

Cut out two cups of tea or coffee.

Stir-fry vegetables, meat or fish, or try dry-frying or use a low-fat oil spray (preferably olive oil).

Eat at least two daily portions of fresh vegetables or fruit – raw, cooked or as salad, as in Day 5.

Drink at least two glasses of water (totalling 500 millilitres, 20 fluid ounces).

Day 3

No more junk food! Swear off especially those foods that contain
E-number artificial additives, always bearing in mind that there
are E-numbers and E- numbers. For instance, avoid the obvious
additives such as the yellow dye tartrazine, which is linked to
ADHD (attention deficit hyperactivity disorder) in children, and
Sudan Red, recently linked with cancer scares. At this stage of the
countdown, don't worry too much about additives such as vitamin
E and ascorbic acid (vitamin C).

Also start avoiding foods with a high sodium and sugar content.
Cut down on both total fat and saturated fat content.

Reduce cola drinks to a single 250 millilitres (10 fluid ounces) glass.

Reduce alcohol consumption to a single unit, preferably diluted
with mineral water (for instance, a white wine spritzer which is
half-and-half, or a single pub measure of vodka with tomato juice).

Confine yourself to a single cup of tea or coffee. Make it weaker
than usual (less caffeine so reduced cravings during detox).

As in Day 4, stir-fry vegetables, meat or fish, or try dry-frying or
use a low-fat oil spray (preferably olive oil). Reduce your fat intake
in other ways: use less butter and mix it half-and-half with a cold-
pressed vegetable spread (cold-pressed usually refers to olive oil
but is also used to prepare other oils like sunflower and corn oil).

Vary the 'bread' part of your meal – experiment with rice cakes, oat
cakes, wholewheat crackers, and start substituting whole-meal
or granary bread for sliced white. Westphalian rye bread –
pumpernickel – is a delicious and healthy alternative.

Make sandwiches using a slice of your usual white and a slice of
healthier granary or wholemeal.

Think grains, pulses, legumes, sweet potatoes and other root vegetables in place of potatoes. Try out one or two of the detox
recipes in Part V using these ingredients, and flavour with herbs
and spices as you like. You then have a dish or two at your finger-
tips for use after your detox starts.

Eat at least three portions of fresh vegetables or fruit as in Day 4.

Drink at least 750 millilitres, 30 fluid ounces (three glasses) of
water during the day.

Day 2

Follow the Day 3 regime, except for the following:

- ✔ No more cola drinks are allowed. Replace them with still or sparkling mineral water, with ice, a slice of lemon or lime, or a little fresh fruit juice.

- ✔ No more alcohol is allowed – replace as for cola drinks.

- ✔ No more tea or coffee is allowed. Replace with a substitute such as bouillon, a glass of hot water and slice of lemon, or a substitute such as organic dandelion 'coffee'.

- ✔ Replace spreading butter with a cold-pressed vegetable spread (and use sparingly).

- ✔ Eat at least four portions of fresh vegetables or fruit.

- ✔ Drink at least four glasses (1 litre, 40 fluid ounces) of water.

Day 1

Follow the Day 2 routine, but eat at least five portions of fresh fruit and vegetables, and drink at least five glasses (1.25 litres, 50 fluid ounces) of water.

You are now ready and prepared to start your own, customised detox programme!

Building Your Own Detox Programme

In the following subsections are detailed plans for three different detox programmes – a weekend, a 7-day, and a 14-day detox. In each case, stock up in advance with the foods and drinks you need.

Choose only organic fruit, vegetables, pulses, and so on, herbal or fruit teas which can be taken throughout, mineral water (or filter jug to remove chlorine from tap water), cleansing and balancing supplements, and other items you need in advance. (Refer to Chapter 5, which talks about what foods to eat.)

Ensure that your juicer is working properly, and make some ice cubes using filtered tap or mineral water. Check that you have sufficient filters if using filtered tap water.

Start each day with a glass of hot water with a little freshly squeezed lemon or lime juice. If you dislike hot water, drink your water on the rocks with a slice of lime or lemon and a squeeze of juice.

For your morning snacks choose one or more pieces of fruit, such as banana, apple, pear, or satsuma. In the afternoon, pick fruit again or drink fruit or veg juice such as apple, carrot, apple and berry; or go for crudités with a tsatziki dip (see chapter 16 for the recipe).

Every day throughout detox, take a multivitamin and mineral complex, vitamin C with bioflavonoids, vitamin E and selenium, and zinc. Every day throughout the balancing stage (which follows the cleansing stage – refer to Chapter 4), add zinc and vitamin B complex.

Planning your detox weekend

Your weekend runs from 7.00 a.m. on Saturday until 7.00 a.m. on Monday. Cleansing gets going on Day 1, then tails off on Day 2, when balancing predominates.

Cleansing Day 1

Breakfast: freshly squeezed fruit or vegetable juice of your choice. Fresh fruit and bio yoghurt, try *Melon with Mixed Berries* (add 125 millilitres/5 fluid ounces fresh bio yoghurt) or *Fresh Blueberry Smoothie* (both recipes are in Chapter 13).

Lunch: bowl of soup such as *Simplest Detox Soup,* or *Tomato, Orange and Ginger* (recipes in chapter 14). Cooked brown rice and a salad such as *Fennel, Caper and Parmesan* or *Asparagus and Blood Orange* (get the recipes in chapter 15).

Dinner: fresh fruit or vegetable juice, brown rice *and Stir-Fry Brussels Sprouts* or *Swede Patties* (see Chapter 17 for the recipes).

Cleansing supplements (see Chapter 3): psyllium husks, milk thistle, dandelion root.

Enjoy – lots of rest and relaxation, gentle yoga or a stroll, long, warm bath with lavender oil and an early night.

Balancing Day 2

Breakfast: freshly squeezed fruit or vegetable juice of your choice. Fresh fruit, bio yoghurt and cereal, such as *Really Delicious Porridge* or *Saturday Morning Muesli* (recipes in Chapter 13).

Lunch: bowl of soup such as *Magic Mushroom and Fennel* or *Galvanising Garlic* (see Chapter14 for the recipes). Cooked brown rice and a salad, such as *Almost Instant Warm Beanshoot Salad* or *Spicy Tuna Salad* (Chapter 15 has the recipes).

Dinner: fresh fruit or vegetable juice, brown rice and *Stir-Fry Brussels Sprouts* or *Swede Patties* (see Chapter 17). Follow the recipes exactly as given or substitute, say, green beans for the Brussels sprouts, and sweet potato or parsnip, pumpkin or turnip for the swede in the second recipe. Fresh fruit, as much as you like.

Cleansing Supplements as during Cleansing Day 1 plus balancing supplements of evening primrose oil and Siberian ginseng.

Get lots of rest and relaxation; do some gentle yoga or take a stroll, and have a long, warm bath with lavender oil and get to bed early.

Planning your 7-day detox

Days 1 to 4 are cleansing days; Days 5 to 7 are for balancing.

Days 1 to 4

Breakfast: freshly squeezed fruit or vegetable juice such as carrot, carrot and apple, and carrot and celery. Bio yoghurt with nuts, seeds and chopped fresh fruit such as melon and banana. *Fresh Figs with Yoghurt and Comb Honey* (see Chapter 13).

Lunch: juice, bowl of soup, salad, for example *Nutty Lambs Lettuce with Sesame Dressing, Asparagus and Blood Orange Salad* (see Chapter 15).

Dinner: fresh fruit or vegetable juice, oat cakes and cottage cheese, or a large bowl of soup such as *Clear Soup with Tofu and Wakame* (see Chapter 14). Cooked grains such as couscous or brown basmati rice, dressed with a little balsamic vinegar and a handful of chopped parsley or chives, for example.

Take cleansing supplements (see Chapter 3) such as psyllium husks, milk thistle, and dandelion root.

Enjoy – lots of rest and relaxation, early nights, yoga and/or a gentle walk, beginning with 20–30 minutes and extending by 15 minutes each day. Take comforting warm baths with tea tree or citrus oil.

Days 5 to 7

Breakfast: fresh fruit or veg juice such as orange and tomato, celery, cucumber and beetroot. Whole grain cereal – *Saturday Morning Muesli* or *Really Delicious Porridge*, for example (recipes in Chapter 13). Feel free to add chopped nuts – brazils, walnuts, or almonds – and/or pumpkin or sunflower seeds.

Lunch: large salad such as *Traditional English Salad* or *Scallop, Chicory and Pomegranate* (see Chapter 15). Follow with fresh fruit such as grapes, pineapple, plums, or greengages.

Dinner: crudités and dips such as *Aubergine and Hazelnut* or *Guacamole* (see Chapter 16). Main course: *Chicken Omelette, Spicy Lime Swordfish,* or *Spaghetti with Mussel Sauce* (recipes in Chapter 18). Green salad or lightly cooked mixed vegetables such as broccoli or spring greens. Fresh fruit to follow.

Continue taking the same cleansing supplements as in Days 1 to 4 plus balancing supplements evening primrose oil and Siberian ginseng.

Enjoy – medium amounts of rest and relaxation, some early nights, yoga, and try 10–20 minutes of meditation. Take slightly more vigorous exercise – walking or perhaps swimming – for up to 40 minutes daily. Comforting warm baths, aromatherapy essences of tea tree, sandalwood, rose or ylang ylang.

Planning your 14-day detox

As in the 7-day detox, the first half of your detox programme is concerned with cleansing, followed by balancing and refreshing.

Days 1 to 7

Breakfast: freshly squeezed fruit or vegetable juice such as pineapple, melon, cranberry, blueberry, or cherry. Bio yoghurt with nuts, seeds, and chopped fresh fruit such as melon or banana; or with prunes, soaked overnight in fresh orange juice. *Fresh Figs with Yoghurt and Comb Honey* (see Chapter 13).

Lunch: bowl of soup, small stick of celery with oatcakes and *Tsatziki dip* (see Chapter 16); salad leaves with cottage cheese mixed with cress, chopped spring onions, and radishes; other salad vegetables in season. Fresh fruit.

Dinner: fresh fruit, or vegetable juice, or crudités and *Tapenade, Hummus* or *Guacamole* (see Chapter 16). Fish such as *Smoked Haddock with Broad Beans and Sweetcorn* or *Prawns with Soy Sauce* (see Chapter 18).

Take cleansing supplements such as psyllium husks, milk thistle, and dandelion root supplement. (See Chapter 3 for a complete list.)

Enjoy – lots of rest and relaxation, early nights, yoga and relaxation exercises, simple meditation. Gentle walking or swimming, beginning with 10–20 minutes and extending by 15 minutes daily. Comforting, warm baths, tea tree or citrus oil as candles or to inhale.

Days 8 to 14

Breakfast: fresh fruit or veg juice such as orange and tomato, watermelon, black or white grape, orange, and papaya and mango. Whole grain cereal, such as *Saturday Morning Muesli, Really Delicious Porridge,* or a cooked breakfast such as *Homemade Baked Beans in Tomato Sauce* with whole grain bread, or *Grilled Mushrooms with Goats Cheese, Tomatoes and Herbs* (all recipes in Chapter 13).

Lunch: Soup such as *Essential Celery Soup* (see Chapter 14), brown rice, bulgur wheat or couscous salad made with chopped fresh herbs, balsamic or cider vinegar, finely chopped garlic, steamed okra (ladies' fingers), chopped radishes, spring onions, watercress, mixed nuts and seeds.

Dinner: crudités and dips such as *Aubergine and Hazelnut, Guacamole* (see Chapter 16). Alternatively, one of the recipe soups in Chapter 14. Main course: *Stir-fried Greens, Mushrooms and Cashew Nuts, Chickpea Curry, Mumbles Leek Tart* or other vegetarian choice from the recipes in chapter 17.

Continue taking cleansing supplements and add the balancing supplements evening primrose oil and Siberian ginseng.

Enjoy – some amounts of rest and relaxation, some early nights, yoga, try 10–20 minutes of simple meditation daily. Take slightly more vigorous exercise than in the first week by walking or perhaps swimming for up to 20–30 minutes daily. Comforting warm baths, aromatherapy essences of tea tree, sandalwood, rose or ylang ylang.

Chapter 11

Supplements for Detox

● ●

● ●

*P*eople tend to join one of two camps where dietary supplements are concerned: one camp proclaims that supplements
are a waste of money and in sometimes harmful; the other camp
recognises the benefits of supplements and uses them regularly.

Detox experts, including yours truly, recommend the use of supplements. This is not to say that their detractors are wrong on every
point. Supplements are not a waste of money if they enhance your
health. However, they do you good only if you take them according
to the therapist's (or packet's) instructions, and do so long enough
for their benefits to be felt. This chapter lays out the whys and
wherefores of supplements, and examines how much you need for
the supplements to be most beneficial when you detox.

Supplementing Your Detox Efforts

Detox supplements are not inherently different from the ordinary
supplements you take for your general health. For instance, you
may already take vitamin C every winter to reduce the risks of
colds and flu, or co-enzyme Q10 when suffering from exhaustion.
The two types of supplement I deal with here are 'dietary' supplements such as minerals and vitamins, and herbal remedies.

Supplements such as vitamins, minerals, and trace elements have
many vital actions on the body's working mechanisms (metabolism) while the antioxidants among them strengthen your immune
system. Many vital nutrients (including the antioxidant sort) help
your liver neutralise and eliminate the many toxins with which it
has to deal. This toxic load increases during detox, when you are
expelling more poisonous waste than usual.

Herbal supplements recommended for detox offer unique benefits, which I address in the sections devoted to specific herbs. All tend to help you eliminate toxins and encourage the development of healthy new tissues and cells.

The safety of certain supplements was brought into question by research during the 1990s suggesting that large doses of certain antioxidant vitamins (vitamin C and beta-carotene, for example) can increase the risks of developing the cancers they were supposed to help prevent (lung cancer, in this example). All the same, millions of people continue to take additional vitamins, minerals, and trace elements and remain pleased with the results.

No dependable scientific tests have portrayed cancer risks as being associated with increased intake of antioxidant vitamins – indeed, a number of studies have found the reverse to be true – that vitamin and mineral supplements cut cancer risks. I can only say that I take them myself, and that you have to decide for yourself whether you wish to do so.

Use supplements with their purpose firmly in mind, that is, to *supplement* your normal, everyday diet. They would indeed be superfluous if your diet always provided all the nutrients you require, magically adjusting to your increased needs when detoxing, say, or suffering a minor infection. This, however, is not the case, and I can wholeheartedly recommend that you use some of the supplements discussed in this book, both during your detox programme and afterwards as the need arises.

For the sake of convenience, herbal remedies are included under the general title of 'supplements'; but you need to remember that many herbs are medicines in their own right, as I indicate under the various headings.

Identifying Your Detox Needs

Detox, like other holistic therapies, emphasises treating the whole person as an individual with unique physical, metabolic, and emotional needs. This means that you take care of your body by removing toxins, and take care of your mind and soul (or emotions, if you prefer) with calmness-inducing relaxation and advice about such issues as relationships and stress management.

Certain supplements – such as vitamin C, selenium, and Coenzyme Q10 – are likely to be useful to most, if not all, detoxers, because of their antioxidant power against free radicals (the hyperactive oxygen molecules that give rise to tissue damage and weaken the immune system). Reading through the information about each kind described below should help you to decide whether it is right for you.

All herbal remedies are plant extracts. They save you from having to chew on platefuls of plants such as milk thistle or globe artichokes (which aren't to everyone's taste). If you do like them, eat artichoke bottoms by all means, but some of the health-giving ingredients may be destroyed by cooking (you can't eat them raw!), and they would be delivering an entirely unknown quantity of helpful ingredients, as opposed to standardised herbal medical preparations.

Camomile is especially helpful if you suffer from insomnia, stress, and/or nervous tension (symptoms of which can be temporarily increased by a stringent detox). Milk thistle may be your best friend if you've drunk too much alcohol in the past and are keen to stop – and hopefully reverse – any liver damage. You may choose globe artichoke if you enjoy eating this vegetable and want to include as many legitimate treats as possible to get you through detox. Corn silk is useful if you periodically suffer from cystitis, an inflammation of the bladder, and want to keep your urinary tract as fit and functional as possible.

Making the Most of Milk Thistle

The herbal supplement supreme to take when you're detoxing is milk thistle (*Silybum marianum*). Milk thistle contains a range of *phytochemicals* (health-promoting plant constituents or ingredients) that benefit the liver. The chiefs of phytochemicals are bioflavonoids, which are highly active antioxidants found in nature in combination with vitamin C. One of the problems of laboratory-produced vitamin C is the absence of bioflavonoids, so you should always look for a natural supplement derived from acerola cherries or rosehips, for example, and check that the bioflavonoids are all present and correct! A good source is silymarin (which has at least 200 times the antioxidant oomph of vitamin C), and silibinin. Many studies have shown that silymarin helps protect liver cells when they're attacked by alcohol, medical chemotherapy, and even death-cap mushrooms. You can read about this, including milk thistle's actions on the body cells, in Chapter 3.

What milk thistle does

Milk thistle is a valuable detox aid and a useful tonic if you drink alcohol regularly or lead a toxic, 21st-century lifestyle with a lot of stress.

This is what milk thistle can do for you:

- Stimulates bile secretion, which helps the gall bladder get rid of toxins and bodily wastes

- Slows down the entry of toxins into liver cells. (This allows the liver to deal with poisons at its own pace instead of becoming overwhelmed by too many at once.)

- Boosts levels of glutathione, the liver's own super-oxidant, which mops up free radicals

- Reduces scar tissue formation which follows when the liver is damaged by repeated toxic overloads. (This can help if you've suffered from a liver disease such as alcoholic cirrhosis or hepatitis, or one of the many kinds of jaundice.)

- Encourages the growth of new liver cells to replace damaged ones when you detox. (Follow this up by living more healthily, by drinking less alcohol, for instance.)

How to take milk thistle

When buying milk thistle capsules, check the silymarin content. For detox purposes, take two capsules each containing 120 milligram silymarin three times daily. For liver protection, which is advisable if you've drunk heavily or live a toxic lifestyle) take two 120 milligram capsules twice daily, preferably between meals. Liver function can start to pick up within as little as five days.

Milk thistle has few reported side-effects. The most common is a mild looseness of the bowels.

If you suffer from gallstones or active (currently being treated) liver disease, take milk thistle only under the guidance of a medical doctor or qualified medical herbalist. This is because milk thistle stimulates bile secretion, and an increased bile volume may not be desirable in your particular case.

Asking for Globe Artichoke

Another member of the thistle family, the globe artichoke (*Cynara scolymus*) provides a healthy snack, light meal, or detox dinner starter, especially when entertaining.

Its physically active ingredients include caffeoylquinic acids, a group of compounds known as 'bitters', which promote digestion, and the potent bioflavonoids inulin, scolymoside, and taraxasterol.

What globe artichoke does

Globe artichoke leaf extract promotes:

- ✔ Bile formation and secretion, which increases the elimination of toxins and body wastes
- ✔ Regeneration of new liver cells to replace damaged ones.

How to take globe artichoke

Eat fresh, lightly-cooked globe artichokes whenever available. Choose heavy, tightly-packed specimens with dark-green leaves.

You can also make a tea of the dried leaves, in which case the recommended amount is 2 grams of dried leaf three times daily.

The recommended dose is a 500 microgram capsule containing 15 milligrams of caffeoylquinic acids two to three times daily.

Globe artichoke is considered a safe medicinal herb with few reported side effects. However, it can produce a severe allergic response in a small number of people, so take it with care if you are prone to dietary allergies.

De-tasselling Corn Silk

Corn silk, the beautiful, pale-green filaments or tassels hidden inside the outer leaves of sweet corn, is known botanically as *Zea mays*, a name befitting a corn goddess!

Corn silk's many phytochemicals include saponins, which act as a diuretic (increasing urine output); thymol, an antiseptic; and the bioflavonoid limonene, a powerful antioxidant that combats the harmful effects of toxins passing through the urinary tract and promotes healthy cell growth.

What corn silk does

Corn silk promotes the detox process by

- ✔ Boosting urinary function, which improves the excretion of water-soluble toxins and encourages the healthy function of the kidneys and bladder
- ✔ Relieving prostate-gland disorders (which impede urine flow and therefore toxin expulsion)

✔ Cleansing the urinary tract of debris, toxins, and surplus mucus, and helping to ward off kidney and bladder infections.

How to take corn silk

You can make a tea of the dried tassels, in which case the recommended dose is 2 to 8 grams, two or three times a day.

You can find corn silk in various herbal remedies for fluid retention and a healthy urinary tract. Take according to label instructions.

Calming Down with Camomile

You may think of camomile in terms of its calming and sedative effect, but this herb also has useful diuretic properties. Its active constituents include salicylate (aspirin-like) derivatives, valerianic acid (also present in the sleep-inducing herb valerian), and antioxidant bioflavonoids such as quercetin and rutin.

What camomile does

As a diuretic, camomile stimulates the flow of urine, helping to rid the body of water-soluble toxins. It also combats inflammation, keeping the bladder, kidneys, and other excretory organs working effectively, and it fights the adverse effects of free radicals.

You can also use camomile to soothe your frayed nerves and help induce a calm, restorative sleep.

How to take camomile

Camomile is readily available from health food stores as dried flower heads, or you can pick the flowers yourself and dry them for personal use.

The recommended dose of camomile in this form is 1 to 4 grams of flower heads taken twice daily plus half-an-hour before retiring for the night.

Supplement:

Take 2–3 g of camomile, in capsules or tablet form, three times daily between meals. Or 1–2 capsules each containing 300–400mg chamomile plant extract, also three times daily between meals.

Do not use camomile for long periods (for instance, for more than three months at a stretch). You may develop an allergy to ragweed (a similar plant) as a result. Use with caution if you are allergic to ragweed, and never use with alcohol or sedatives.

Spreading Evening Primrose Oil

This plant seed extract is a rich source of the omega-6 nutrient gammalinolenic acid. Your body manufactures gammalinolenic acid from cis-linoleic acid found in cold-pressed vegetable oils such as rapeseed and safflower. However, factors such as ageing, viruses, consuming unhealthy trans-fats in junk food, and ultra-violet rays can interfere with this process, leaving you short of hormone-like prostaglandins needed for the minute-by-minute control of skin cells and other bodily systems.

What evening primrose oil does

Skin, like the other eliminatory organs, works best when in good condition. Clean, healthy skin exudes perspiration (and toxins) more freely.

Sore, inflamed patches of skin are a deterrent to skin brushing, which consists of brushing the skin all over your body with the exception of your face, genitals, and perineum (the area between your genitals and the anus). As an adjunct to detox, you can skin brush yourself once a day, for example, using a loofah or other suitable bristle brush (nothing too scratchy or harsh!) Carry this out before showering or bathing, as the toxins brought to the surface can then be rinsed away as you wash.

Evening primrose oil (EPO) enhances the health and vitality of skin (and hair and nails), by:

- Helping it to shed dead cells and regenerate new ones
- Combating inflammatory skin conditions such as eczema and psoriasis
- Maintaining the skin's natural oil content, thereby combating dry, rough skin
- Boosting the immune defence system, helping to fight skin infections and age-related wrinkles
- Easing the pain and stiffness of inflammatory joint conditions such as rheumatoid and osteo-arthritis.

How to take evening primrose oil

Take two to three 500 milligram capsules daily during detox, and perhaps one or two daily thereafter. Alternatively, soften the capsules in a little warm water and apply the resulting paste to dry, roughened, and inflamed skin. The oil is available in small quantities but doesn't taste nice and is much more expensive than buying capsules.

EPO is generally safe to take, but caution is needed if you suffer from epilepsy or other types of convulsions. One study carried out during the 1980–90s, in which people with epilepsy took EPO, suggested an increased tendency to epileptic seizures.

Spicing Things Up with Cayenne

A hot, red spice made from a range of chilli peppers, the capsaicin in cayenne helps you eliminate toxins through your skin by making you sweat. Other useful nutrients include antioxidant bioflavonoids that combat the harmful effect of free radicals and ascorbic acid (vitamin C, another powerful antioxidant).

What cayenne does

Cayenne is a strong circulatory stimulant, increasing the blood flow through all areas of your body, (thereby accelerating toxin release), which in turn increases the formation of sweat.

Cayenne also provides a vitamin-like active ingredient with antioxidant functions, to combat free radical damage. It also flushes out diseased tissue cells and helps to reverse early stages of degenerative disorders (such as ageing changes) and chronic inflammation (such as in arthritis).

How to take cayenne

You can easily add cayenne to food – many savoury dishes benefit from a little 'spicing up'. You can also add a pinch to freshly prepared juices such as carrot, cucumber, celery, apple, and tomato.

Do not use cayenne if you suffer from an acid stomach, and do not apply it directly to mucous membranes such as the lining of the mouth or other areas. Its 'burning' quality may aggravate a tender stomach lining, and cause great soreness to delicate mucous membranes.

Picking Dandelion

Botanically known as *Taraxacum officinalis*, dandelion's springtime leaves have been prized for centuries as the base for a herbal tonic, and its roots (especially those of two-year-old plants) have beneficial all-round detoxifying properties. These two main actions are not entirely confined to the leaves and roots but are largely concentrated here. Adding a few leaves to a salad provides a good source of nutrients and tonic effects. Roots are also good in salads.

What dandelion does

Dandelion aids liver cleansing by stimulating its detoxifying functions, including bile flow which boosts the elimination of toxic waste by the intestines. It also acts as diuretic, promoting urine, which helps you eliminate water-soluble toxins.

Dandelion cleanses the blood, promoting the destruction of ageing blood cells and the production of new replacements. It also improves the function of the kidneys (eliminating water-soluble toxins); the pancreas (enhancing digestive tract function and the elimination of toxins by the gut); the spleen (and therefore the activity of the toxin-combating immune defence system); and the stomach (important to the efficient function of the gut and the elimination of gut toxins).

How to take dandelion

Add fresh young dandelion leaves or freshly sliced root to salads, making sure that you pick the greens only from unpolluted sites.

Take 5 to 10 grams of fresh root daily in divided doses (2-year-old plants are recommended), or a 500 milligram extract twice daily.

If you have gallstones, take dandelion only under qualified medical or herbal supervision. Dandelion should be avoided during an acute gallstones attack (known medically as cholecystitis) and other forms of obstructive jaundice. Dandelion stimulates the production of bile, which would be undesirable during an attack, as the gall bladder is in an inflamed condition.

Taking Your Vitamin B Complex

Your liver needs water-soluble B-group vitamins to produce energy and to help process alcohol and other toxins. Collectively, B vitamins release energy during the metabolic breakdown of fats, carbohydrates, and proteins and are vital both to the liver and, less obviously, to other excretory organs for on-going supplies of energy.

Stress and a high alcohol intake both deplete B complex vitamin stores, which can directly affect liver function and toxin excretion.

What vitamin B does

B complex as a whole encourages healthy metabolism and reduces the ill effects of stress on the body. The detox-related functions of three of the B vitamin group are:

- ✔ Thiamine (B1) helps with energy production (vital during detox) and with the proper function of your gut, liver, and central nervous system. Thiamine is also an antioxidant, and protects the liver and other organs from both the ageing process and the toxins supplied to the body in cigarette smoke and alcohol.

- ✔ Riboflavin (B2) boosts antibody production by the immune defence system, and energy production through the metabolism of carbohydrates, fats, and proteins. You need energy while detoxing, and a major aim of your all-over cleansing is to reinvigorate your immune system.

Your eating regimen while detoxing is limited to specific foods, which means that you need to derive the maximum energy and nutritional benefit from meals at this time. Riboflavin can help you in this respect, but is easily destroyed by antibiotics and alcohol, and you need extra when stressed or undertaking strenuous physical work or exercise.

- ✔ Pantothenic acid (B5) is *the* anti-stress vitamin; it is important in the production of fight-or-flight hormones – adrenaline and noradrenaline – and of antibodies by the immune system. Many detoxers suffer from stress, and the regimen itself poses certain challenges due to lifestyle and dietary change.

Pantothenic acid also helps your body utilise other vitamins supplied by the diet or supplements, and boosts the production of energy from dietary fats, carbohydrates and proteins.

Pantothenic acid has a protective effect on liver cells even when the cells are overwhelmed by viral toxins, produced by viruses. When 150 viral hepatitis sufferers took B5 supplements, their liver function tests improved significantly, and they made more antibodies, fighting the infection more effectively.

How to take vitamin B complex

B vitamin complex comes as capsule and tablets. Buy a reputable brand in which the majority of Bs included are of 50 milligram strength, and follow the directions on the label carefully.

Mooning over Selenium

Selenium, named after the Greek moon goddess, is found in plants grown on soil rich in this mineral. Selenium in the soil is uncommon in Europe hence European plants do not, on the whole, contain much selenium. It occurs more frequently in the Americas.

What selenium does

Selenium subdues harmful reactions within the liver sparked by ongoing toxin processing. It also enhances the activities of the liver enzyme P450, which deals with toxins, and helps to repair damaged genetic material. Furthermore, selenium helps to protect you from liver cancer sparked by the huge toxic overload with which this organ frequently deals.

How to take selenium

Take 100 to 200 micrograms of selenium daily during detox. After your detox consider continuing to do so for life.

You can safely take up to 450 micrograms daily but toxicity can occur above 800 micrograms daily. Signs of selenium toxicity include a garlicky body odour, blackened or fragile fingernails, a metallic taste in the mouth, nausea, dizziness, and hair loss. This is not life-threatening, merely undesirable and unpleasant.

Chapter 12

Maintaining Detox for Life

*T*his chapter shows you how you can use the principles of detox for the rest of your life. Why lose the benefits of going back to your old, toxic way of eating and living?

Keeping It Going

Keeping it going does not mean detoxing forever! It simply means incorporating detox principles into your diet and lifestyle, together with plenty of sources of fun and pleasure. It's not about denying yourself, but about striking a happy and healthy balance.

Here are some points to consider as your detox approaches its end.

Focusing on food

Don't be tempted to celebrate your successful detox by bingeing on the foods you perhaps fantasised about while detoxing. Heading straight for the pub or ordering a heavy, greasy takeaway meal may well upset your stomach and would certainly overload your system with toxins you worked hard to expel.

Be kind to your liver, kidneys, lungs, gut, and skin – that is, be kind to yourself! Re-introduce less digestible foods such as bread (especially white), red meat, full-fat cheese, fried and roast dishes, and alcohol, over 1–2 weeks in gradually increasing amounts.

Keep with the organic! Even a weekend detox puts you in touch with local sources of organic fruit and vegetables; a 7- or 14-day detox means several trips out to replenish your stocks of organic produce and meat. (Refer to Chapter 10, which explains how to do short, medium, and long detoxes.) I am sure you'll notice the superior flavour of organic foods, and you can comfort yourself for their greater cost by remembering their nutritional benefits, and freedom from artificial growing agents. Continue, also, to buy organic bread, biscuits, frozen vegetarian dishes, dried fruit, nuts and seeds, pulses, grains, and pasta.

You can also start making more of your own dishes, especially if you relied heavily on pre-packaged convenience foods in the past. Spend a weekend afternoon, every two to three weeks, cooking and freezing delectable, healthy dishes. You could even form a small co-operative with one or more friends, agreeing on menus and exchanging frozen foods you each enjoy cooking – and eating!

Regular treats are also a must, even if forbidden during detox. Chocolate, containing mood-boosting theobromine, springs to mind – eat it occasionally, choosing the dark, gleaming, expensive sort with a cocoa mass of 70 per cent or more. A little cocoa-rich chocolate, with its subtle bouquet and flavour, soon satisfies. Other random treats include tahini, the sesame paste used to make hummus. Blended with fresh lime or lemon juice and a little water, it makes an excellent salad dressing. You can also try the nut butters – hazelnut, cashew nut, almond, brazil, macadamia – that make delicious dips and spreads.

You can find many satisfying and healthy recipes in vegetarian cookbooks. Include vegetarian dishes in your normal meat- and fish-based eating plans, or be adventurous and designate a day or so every week for vegetarian eating.

Tapping into your fluids

Keeping your fluids in balance is an important part of maintaining your detox lifestyle. Pouring in the water helps your organs cleanse and stay hydrated. Caffeine, carbonation, and alcohol can counter water's benefits and introduce toxins as well, so you want to avoid those liquids.

Guzzling water

One of the most important habits to continue after detoxing is that of drinking at least eight glasses (250 millilitres, 10 fluid ounces) of water every day. Though a fairly simple thing to do during a dedicated detox, eight glasses can seem a tall order when back to everyday life.

Use the following tips to organise eight glasses of water into your daily routine:

✔ Make full use of any water cooler/heater supplied at work.

✔ Now that 500 millilitre bottles of mineral water are trendy, take a few to work and store in the fridge, keep a couple in your handbag or briefcase, sip watching TV or reading at home, or when working, travelling, exercising, relaxing . . . whenever.

✔ Make things interesting for yourself – alternate cool bottled mineral water with hot water (mineral or filtered tap). Flavour hot or cold water with a freshly cut slice of lime or lemon, or use sachets to turn the hot water into herbal, flower, or fruit tea.

Pulling back from caffeine and alcohol

Go easy on tea and coffee to reduce your intake of addictive caffeine, which boosts urine formation and encourages dehydration.

Keep any alcohol consumption within safe limits – 14 units weekly for a woman, 21 for a man. A 175 millilitre glass of wine or a pint of ordinary strength lager is two units (strong lager is three units), a pub measure of spirits is one unit.

Keeping to this limit may seem easier said than done, but a few simple measures can help:

✔ Decide how much you are going to drink before joining friends for a meal or pub session.

✔ Never drink on an empty stomach – a sudden alcohol hit to the brain can banish your best laid plans.

✔ Buy your own drinks, rather than rounds. It gives you more control.

✔ Alternate glasses of water with glasses of wine, beer, or spirits.

✔ Choose a low-alcohol wine or beer for a change, and dilute wine or spirits with healthy mixers such as sparkling mineral water, tomato juice, or soda water.

Do an assertiveness course if you don't like to be seen curbing your drinking! It's *your* liver you just detoxed and *your* health that is at stake.

If it's really impossible for you to spend an evening with hard-drinking friends while abstaining yourself, then frankly you're better off avoiding the hassle altogether.

Choose an alternative to a night in the pub or wine bar (no, you *don't* have to spend it exercising!). Join an evening class, take up watercolour painting or take your Advanced Driver's Test.

Moving into exercise

Regular gentle exercise creates a need for itself! After just two days of detox, you're likely to miss the benefits of stretching and bending, simple yoga poses, and walking. Set aside a few minutes every day to continue with this gentle exercise, varying the length of time and the variety of exercise to avoid monotony.

More demanding exercise also becomes addictive! It may be hard at first to persuade yourself to do 20 minutes on a treadmill or exercise bicycle, go for a brisk walk or swim a few lengths of a pool. But your reward will be twofold in that you gain a great sense of achievement (keep a chart, if it helps, and tick off your planned aerobic exercise sessions), and you slash the risks of obesity, heart attacks and strokes, lower your blood pressure, and help maintain a healthy cholesterol level.

What's more, exercise improves your blood circulation, which brings extra oxygen to your tissues to fight toxic free radicals (the hyperactive oxygen molecules which harm your immune system and other organs). In addition, your stress levels subside, further limiting the formation of free radicals.

Making way for relaxation

If, before your detox, you were unused to 'real' relaxation, you'll realise how beneficial it can be. (Refer to Chapter 9, which offers relaxation tips and techniques.) Relaxation is a huge stress-beater (and therefore demolisher of harmful free radicals). It frees the body of stiffness and muscle tension (as well as many aches, pains, and minor ailments). It also brings a sense of calm: obstacles and dilemmas lose much of their power to scare when your mind and emotions are at peace. You are then empowered to deal with problems more effectively.

However challenging it may seem, aim to take at least twenty minutes every day to sit quietly, practise relaxation (refer to Chapter 9), and listen to calming music or, if possible, meditate.

Getting restful sleep

In his play *Macbeth*, Shakespeare speaks of sleep as the 'balm of hurt minds' and goes on to say that it 'knits up the ravelled sleave of care.' Sleep is, and always has been, a great antidote to trauma and stress, and you need good quality, restful sleep to combat the toxic effects of today's tiresome, stressful world.

Your sleep may be slightly disturbed by detoxing because your body and mind face many new challenges during detox. But its quality should rebalance itself afterwards, or improve in quality in response to a healthier diet and regular exercise and relaxation.

 If you have suffered from insomnia for a long time, see your doctor in case there is an underlying health cause. An overactive thyroid gland, menopausal symptoms, digestive upsets, a weak bladder, anxiety disorders, and clinical depression are just some of the factors that can trigger sleeping problems.

If you have trouble sleeping, try the following simple tips that work for many people:

- ✔ Eliminate potential culprits such as an overheated or draughty bedroom, uncomfortable mattress, noise, and watching scary films before switching off the light.

- ✔ Avoid heavy meals and alcohol in the evening and try a milky drink last thing. You don't have to be an old granny (or granddad) to sip hot milk in bed! The calcium it supplies calms the nerves and helps you relax physically and mentally.

- ✔ Try a herbal remedy such as valerian, which comes as sachets for making into tea (the sachets never fail me, whatever the cause of my unrest). Alternatively, choose a product such as Quiet Life (made by Lanes Health Products Ltd.), which combines valerian with other soporific herbs plus nerve-calming vitamins. Quiet Life is available from most pharmacies and health food shops.

Thinking Long Term

If you follow the guidelines outlined in the preceding section, is there any need to think about your long term health? Barring accidents and surgical emergencies, won't your good health be more or less guaranteed?

Well, no, not precisely. A lot depends upon your *genetic health profile* – the weaknesses and ailment tendencies that run in your family – and upon unforeseen factors over which you have no, or very little, control. Loss of job or partner, money worries, ill health of loved ones, having to move house – these and similar factors can place you under intolerable strain. And stress, of course, can harm your health however carefully you eat, drink, and relax.

The subsections here offer suggestions for you to consider in order to maintain and improve your long-term health.

Doing regular detoxes

How often you detox is your personal choice, depending upon the time you have available. But many regular detoxers complete two or three programmes every year, with single day or weekend detoxes in between. (Chapter 10 outlines DIY detox programmes.) Popular times for detox programmes are early spring, to slough off toxins and excess weight accumulated throughout the winter, and early autumn, to capitalise on the health benefits of summer and boost the immune defence system against winter ills. Many also detox in January, to dispel toxins taken on board over the Christmas season.

You may like to follow this plan, and add a weekend or two in summer and winter, say, if you feel the need. Single day detoxes are an effective way of counteracting an unhealthy, weekend, for instance, or simply a night on the Town.

Scheduling health MOTs

Schedule an annual (or more frequent) general health check. Ask your doctor to answer any queries you have and check essential health parameters. Normally included should be your general health and weight, your blood pressure, blood sugar level, and other blood tests, and an analysis of your urine.

You can easily dovetail your annual health check with a medication review to determine that you're taking the pills you need and aren't taking any that you don't need.

Women, you also need regular cervical smears while you're of child-bearing age and a mammogram twice a year if you're over fifty. Men, if you're fifty or older, you need a PSA (protein-specific antigen) test, which monitors the prostate gland for cancerous changes.

Reviewing your life status

In addition to regular medical MOTs, other checkups, which you can do yourself, also promote long-term health.

Stress plays such a prominent role in generating toxic free radicals that you need to take regular stock of the strain you are under and decide whether you can reduce your load to more tolerable limits.

How often do you need to do take stock? Ideally, each time you follow a detox programme, if you intend to do so several times a year as suggested in the previous section. If not, then assess your stress rating at six monthly intervals, say, and adjust your stress-beating plan accordingly.

I recommend the www.1DO3.com/uk Web site, which provides assessment questionnaires from which you can ascertain your stress level, and www.stressbusting.co.uk , which gives plenty of tips to help you beat your own particular triggers. Other Web sites that can help you assess your stress levels are www.bbc.co.uk/health/tv_and_radio/stresstest_quizindex.shtml, www.internethealthlibrary.com/sq/stress/stress-assess.htm, and www.less-stress.com/

You may also find Chapters 8 and 9 helpful as they explain how to overcome stress and embrace relaxation, respectively. (I especially recommend mastering one of Chapter 8's 'relax in the moment' techniques.)

A dedicated period of complete relaxation daily, helps to cleanse, balance and refresh your mind and body. Events such as bereavement or divorce are universally recognised stress triggers, but it's often the little irritations that cause you to flip your lid (and feel embarrassed or guilty afterwards, which merely compounds the stress).

Just imagine smiling calmly when caught in a traffic jam and late for an appointment, or merely taking deep relaxing breaths after dropping your handbag all over the platform during a rush-hour stampede.

Nourishing with nutritional supplements

Chapter 11 talks about supplements that boost the various stages of detox. Many health-conscious people take baseline supplements year-round, just adding specific cleansing and balancing remedies during their detox programme.

The combinations from which you can choose are almost infinite. I give details here of my personal choice of supplements to boost general health and minimise the damaging effects of free radicals and other toxins:

✔ A high potency multivitamin and mineral combination

✔ Additional vitamin C with bioflavonoids

✔ A magnesium and calcium combination

✔ Evening primrose oil (providing omega-6 fatty acids)

✔ Fish oil extract (providing omega-3 fatty acids)

✔ Lecithin

✔ Blueberry extract

✔ Gingko biloba extract

✔ Siberian ginseng for 2–3 months, during spring and autumn when cold and flu viruses are most common.

Making Little Changes for Big Benefits

Small changes can seem too small to be worth the effort. This may seem especially true if you decided to abolish your unhealthy habits and are going for detox perfection.

Perhaps you set yourself detox goals – such as *never* drinking alcohol again, or *always* exercising for half an hour daily. Then you find yourself unable to achieve what you set out to do. If you're like many people, you become angry – with yourself and with your goals. You start to view detox as unachievable. And the next stop? You return to your toxic habits.

The first thing to realise is that detox perfection doesn't actually exist. Detox is an ongoing process that you adjust to and make adjustments to depending on your body and your circumstances.

Try to see living with fewer toxins as a lifetime goal. For several decades at least, you have eaten unhealthily, and maybe acquired certain toxic habits. Be kind to yourself! You cannot sweep away inbuilt eating and behavioural patterns within a couple of weeks (or months). It takes some people years . . . and that's okay.

Refuse to be discouraged by a few (or numerous) slip-ups. You overate today, then binged on chocolate. Forget it, and continue with your new habits, starting *now*. You can make small changes that achieve real detox benefits. The idea is to make changes as painless (and enjoyable) as possible.

Integrating exercise

If you hate walking (for instance) but walking remains your easiest and most accessible exercise, don't plan lengthy hikes for yourself! Three 10-minute walks a day are in fact more beneficial than one 30-minute one. Plan your day to include such walks, three or four times a week.

Also, use the stairs and not the lift in your workplace, try parking a little further from the shops or your office and catching your bus or train one stop or station down the line. All the above actually work to increase the amount of exercise you get. You may need to stagger your shopping to avoid carrying a load if you park blocks away from the shops, but staggering should encourage you to shop more selectively and buy only the healthy foods you need!

If you'd frankly rather watch telly than stride 'unnecessary' distances, buy an exercise bike! You can then get exercise while viewing your favourite soap.

Freshening your food choices

Aim always to buy organic fruit and veg. Whenever organic proves impossible, buy the freshest-looking ones you can find, and wash them thoroughly to remove agricultural toxins.

Trick your taste buds and appestat (your brain's appetite regulator) into gaining satisfaction from healthy foods. If you're craving fresh dairy cream, substitute Greek-style yoghurt or reduced-fat crème fraiche.

Satisfy a sweet tooth with a teaspoonful of organic honey or maple syrup. Concoct a delicious, filling baguette using the freshest bakery produce available, and fill with mashed avocado in place of mayonnaise, and a handful of fresh or defrosted prawns.

Find other treats to satisfy cravings in the recipe chapters in Part V – build up your own repertoire for use in an emergency!

Part V
Delicious Detox Recipes

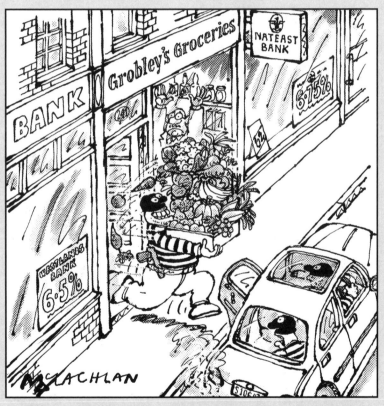

"Butch has never been the same since
he discovered detoxing."

In this part . . .

*H*ere I give you six chapters containing healthy detox recipes using a wide range of delicious ingredients to help you eliminate toxic waste. The recipes range from breakfasts – including ideas for anyone who normally avoids this meal – soups, salads – including a number of fresh and delectable foods you may not have considered eating in salad form before – snacks, dips and spreads – yes, snacks are permissible when detoxing, which means that you need never go hungry again – and main meals based on protein from fish and fowl.

If you're a vegetarian there's recipes for you, too. Many of the recipes are suitable for vegetarians but there's also a chapter dedicated to vegetarians wanting to detox.

Chapter 13

Detox Breakfasts

In This Chapter

▶ Making food choices to start your detox day

▶ Preparing breakfast recipes

*B*reakfast is often said to be the most important meal of the day (even if it's rarely the most popular). This is because starting a day 'on empty' (compare your body to a car running low on petrol!) means starting off your morning at a nutritional and energy-linked disadvantage compared to regular breakfasters. This is not the way to get, or to give, the most your day has to offer.

Starting Your Detoxing Day Off Right

Whatever you're aim, getting your day off to a good start augurs well for satisfaction later on. Here you will learn about the importance of breakfast when detoxing, and the foods both to choose and to avoid!

Breaking your fast with good foods

Breaking your fast when you are detoxing is even more important – you have been eating less than usual, probably of foods that you've seldom sampled before. Your body is also working hard, firstly disposing of toxins, then rebalancing and re-energising itself.

You'll probably feel the need of something substantial – porridge, home-made baked beans in tomato sauce, and muesli would all fit the bill. They are based on low-G.I. carbohydrates to give you a vitality boost and to calm hunger pangs.

If something lighter takes your fancy, try the exotic fruit platter, yoghurt with banana and walnuts or a fresh berry smoothie. All three provide antioxidant-rich fruit with fairly low G.I. to give you a lift without a 'glucose high' (when your blood sugar soars skyward, then plummets into your boots, leaving you exhausted and shaky).

Nuts supply energy and some protein, as well as a little oil and, undoubtedly for nut lovers, satisfying texture and flavour. (They're also quite filling!)

The milk and/or bio-yoghurt in the yoghurt and smoothie provide calcium and other minerals for well-being and strong bones, while the helpful bacteria in the bio-yoghurt cleanses and balances your hard-working gut.

In fact, here's a list of the benefits you can find in the breakfast recipes included in this chapter.

Steering clear of non-starters

If you do eat breakfast (but not exactly healthily), now is the time to kick cupboard culprits into touch! You need to avoid processed food laden with E-numbers, such as sugary cereals, sugary fruit juices, and sugary smoothies, because the whole purpose of detox is to release stored toxins resulting from such items. They are also high G.I., and give you an energy kick, followed soon afterwards with a low-energy state.

For the same reason, white bread is out, as are sugar and whole-fat milk added to your drinks and low G.I. cereals. After a while, you will find how much better you feel eating detox foods in place of the chocolate bar you usually nibble on the way to work, or the greasy sausages, bacon, and fried bread with which you've started each day.

Banana Yoghurt with Walnuts

This recipe is filling, delicious, and light. There's plenty of potassium in the banana to help combat bloating, and the bio-yoghurt eases any gut discomfort while encouraging its cleansing action.

Preparation time: *1 minute*

Serves: *1*

6–7 tablespoons (tablespoon) plain bio-yoghurt, chilled overnight

1 banana, sliced into chunks

1 tablespoon chopped walnuts

Cinnamon to taste

1 Mix the chopped banana and the yoghurt, scatter with the chopped walnut and season to taste with the powdered cinnamon.

> ***Per serving:*** *Calories 214 (From Fat 76); Fat 9 g (Saturated 3 g); Cholesterol 12 mg; Sodium 44 mg; Carbohydrate 33 g (Dietary Fibre 4 g); Protein 6 g.*

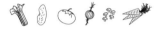

Fresh Blueberry Smoothie

How delicious, to start the day with a fresh fruit smoothie! Use any soft fruit you like – blueberries are a great favourite with smoothie fans, as their flavour is as great as their nutritional benefits (they are amazingly high in antioxidants and powerfully good for small blood vessels).

You can also make a blueberry smoothie using frozen berries. Either way, your breakfast drink is providing one of your five fruit and veg portions for the day.

Preparation time: *5 minutes*

Serves: *1*

Large handful of fresh blueberries

1 fresh mango, peeled, pitted and chopped

Six ice cubes

Freshly squeezed orange juice (optional)

1 teaspoon (teaspoon) organic honey (optional)

1 heaped desserteaspoonoon (dsp) thick bio yoghurt

Fresh mint leaves for decoration

(continued)

(continued)

1 Use a smoothie maker, a blender or a food processor. Whizz the blueberries, mango, and ice cubes together, and add a little freshly squeezed orange juice to reach desired consistency. If the mango is very ripe, you may need only a little extra juice.

2 Taste the smoothie, and sweeten with the honey if required.

3 Float the yoghurt on the surface and decorate with fresh mint leaves.

Use warm thick honey for easy stirring.

Frozen blueberries retain a high percentage of their original nutrients.

Per serving: Calories 184 (From Fat 13); Fat 1 g (Saturated 0 g); Cholesterol 1 mg; Sodium 7 mg; Carbohydrate 45 g (Dietary Fibre 4 g); Protein 1 g.

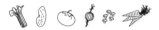

Saturday Morning Muesli

I called this Saturday morning muesli because, if you make it fresh each time, amalgamating all the ingredients may be more than you have time for before leaving for school, work or weekday shopping.

However, you can make up the dry ingredients once a week and store the muesli in air-tight containers.

You can use other cereal crops – flaked rye, barley or wheat, for instance. But there's something especially comforting about the flavour and texture of fresh oat flakes, and they are recognised, prime soothers of mind and nerves.

Preparation time: *Overnight + 3 minutes*

Serves: *1*

2 heaped tablespoon of flaked porridge oats

2 heaped tablespoon of oat bran

½ fresh apple or pear, grated or chopped

1 dsp sultanas or raisins or dried currants

Few curls of grated fresh coconut

1 level teaspoon poppy seeds

3 tablespoon bio-yoghurt or 250 ml reduced fat goats milk

¼– ½ teaspoon freshly ground nutmeg

1 Soak the oat flakes, bran, and dried fruit overnight in a little pure water or yoghurt/milk. First thing, mix the soaked ingredients together with the apple and any juice, and the yoghurt or milk. Stir in the coconut flakes. Scatter with poppy seeds and nutmeg.

Coconut's fat is primarily saturated, but a small amount is acceptable, and it adds other essential nutrients and a great flavour. 'Saturday morning' muesli uses more ingredients than you may have time to assemble on weekdays. But enjoy it whenever you fancy!

Per serving: Calories 175 (From Fat 70); Fat 8 g (Saturated 5 g); Cholesterol 0 mg; Sodium 6 mg; Carbohydrate 29 g (Dietary Fibre 6 g); Protein 5 g.

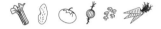

Jewelled Pink Grapefruit

I cannot resist including this recipe in *Detox For Dummies* although I warn against drinking actual grapefruit juice during a detox in Chapter 3 (Supporting Your Detox Organs). Its freshness and delightful appearance cheer the gloomiest morning, so choose it as a breakfast treat on the final day of a short detox or during the last three days of a 7- or 14- day detox programme, when your body is busy refreshing itself.

Preparation time: *10 minutes*

Serves: *1*

1 grapefruit	*1–2 teaspoon honey*
1–2 tablespoon pomegranate seeds	*Fresh mint leaves for decoration*

1 Cut your grapefruit in half and prepare one or both halves depending upon your early morning appetite. Separate the flesh from the surrounding membrane and pith, and use a teaspoon to widen some of the gaps surrounding the segments. Slide the pomegranate seeds down into the gaps, and scatter any remaining seeds over the surface of the fruit. Reserve any juice produced.

2 Drizzle with the honey and place under a hot grill for 2–3 minutes, depending upon the grill's heat. Watch its progress constantly – you want hot fruit with slightly caramelised honey, you do not want it burned to charcoal black. Remove from the heat, spoon over reserved juice, and decorate with fresh mint leaves.

(continued)

(continued)

A little grapefruit is safe enough but refer to Chapter 3, which tells you why you don't want to eat too much.

Honey – organic nutrients are bactericidal and slow down absorption of natural sugar, minimising 'sugar rush'.

Per serving: Calories 105 (From Fat 0); Fat 0 g (Saturated 0 g); Cholesterol 0 mg; Sodium 1 mg; Carbohydrate 27 g (Dietary Fibre 4 g); Protein 2 g.

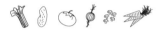

Exotic Fruit Platter

For a touch of the exotic in your detox try this delicious fruit-filled recipe. It's a quick and lovely treat.

Preparation time: *5 minutes*

Serves: *1*

Slices of paw paw (papaya), mango, lychees, pomegranate, and Chinese gooseberries (kiwi fruit)	Bio-yoghurt for dipping
	Powdered Ginger
	Caraway seeds

1 Wash and slice as many fruits as you fancy or can obtain. Pat fruit slices dry, arrange them on a large platter and season with powdered ginger. Shake a few caraway seeds over the bio-yogurt and drizzle with a little warmed organic honey. Dip fruit slices into the yoghurt. You can also use this breakfast recipe for a dessert, giving guests forks to spear the fruit pieces.

Per serving: Calories 198 (From Fat 40); Fat 4 g (Saturated 3 g); Cholesterol 16 mg; Sodium 61 mg; Carbohydrate 37 g (Dietary Fibre 2 g); Protein 5 g.

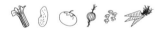

Homemade Baked Beans in Tomato Sauce

Are you surprised that you can actually enjoy 'beans on toast' during your detox? Well, you shouldn't be! Beans and pulses are prime suppliers of low-G.I. ingredients, and tomatoes are 'top of the pops' for sheer antioxidant power and cancer-fighting properties. Homemade beans on toast are also, incidentally, far more delicious than the commercial kind – not to mention being chock-full of great nutritional benefits.

Preparation time: *20 minutes*

Serves: *2–3*

1 medium onion, sliced

1–2 teaspoon olive oil

4 medium tomatoes, chopped

1–2 tablespoon tomato puree

½ teaspoon mixed dried herbs

Large pinch mustard powder

1 tablespoon soy sauce

1 450 gram (15 ounce) can of haricot or red kidney beans, drained

1 heaped teaspoon molasses or dark-brown soft sugar

150 ml (¼ pint) water

1 Fry onion in oil in covered pan until soft. Add the tomatoes, tomato puree and water, bring to the boil, then simmer gently for 7–10 minutes until soft. Stir in the herbs, mustard powder, soy sauce, and molasses or sugar. When it has cooled slightly, whizz the sauce in a blender and return it to the pan with the beans. Cook over a low heat for 5 minutes. Serve on (or with) toasted slices of sour dough or whole-wheat bread.

If you don't feel like peeling a large onion, top and tail 3–4 spring onions instead, and cut them into chunks.

Molasses is a traditional ingredient of American baked bean recipes, but omit it if you like, or substitute a heaped teaspoon of dark-brown soft sugar.

Per serving: *Calories 242 (From Fat 30); Fat 3 g (Saturated 0 g); Cholesterol 0 mg; Sodium 854 mg; Carbohydrate 42 g (Dietary Fibre 9 g); Protein 13 g.*

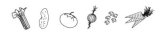

Grilled Mushrooms with Goat's Cheese, Tomatoes, and Herbs

How delicious is goat's cheese! If you eat cheese and have never tried it, here is your chance! It has an insistent, though mild, flavour, and goes so well with a wide range of accompanying ingredients such as breads and biscuits, tomatoes, mushrooms, and nearly all vegetables. In fact, goat's cheese is quite addictive! And *extremely* good for you...

Preparation time: *13 minutes*

Serves: *1*

2 large open-cap mushrooms

2 heaped dsp soft/reduced fat goats cheese

1–2 tomatoes, sliced

1–2 tablespoons olive oil

Handful chopped basil

Freshly ground black pepper

1 Tear basil into pieces. Arrange tomato slices on a large plate, scatter the basil over the slices and drizzle very lightly with olive oil, if liked.

2 Wipe the mushrooms and remove their stalks. Lightly brush mushroom caps all over with the oil, chop up the stalks, and mix them with the goats cheese. Season with black pepper. Fill the inverted mushroom cups with the cheese mixture, and cook under a medium grill for 5–10 minutes, checking frequently to avoid burning. Serve hot and melting, with the tomato and basil salad.

Per serving: Calories 215 (From Fat 140); Fat 16 g (Saturated 3 g); Cholesterol 3 mg; Sodium 77 mg; Carbohydrate 12 g (Dietary Fibre 2 g); Protein 3 g.

Fresh Figs with Yoghurt and Comb Honey

Could anything be more delicious than the breakfast (or lunch) the Greeks have enjoyed since time immemorial? Yoghurt provides you with calcium plus the sheer deliciousness and cosseting you need to start each day. Comb honey is obtainable if you look around a little. Bee-keepers usually have some for sale, as do superior food stores such as Harrods, Selfridges, Fortnum and Mason, and others online.

Figs you may recognise from childhood and have unfriendly memories. Forget syrup of figs (a laxative) and the hard, chewy items once representing figs in their dried state. You can now buy the 'dried' item (when you cannot find the fresh version, of course) as succulent, delicious, semi-dried fruit in nearly all supermarkets.

You can use cow's or goat's yoghurt, but the goat variety makes this Greek recipe just that little bit more authentic.

Preparation time: *2 minutes*

Serves: *1*

2–3 fresh ripe figs	*Fresh honeycomb*
4–5 tablespoon bio-yoghurt (cow's milk or goat's milk)	*Cinnamon to taste*

You barely need a recipe for this sunshine breakfast, widely eaten in Peloponnese mountain villages in Greece.

1 Halve the figs, and arrange these beautiful objects on your best plate. Sprinkle with a little cinnamon, and spoon the thick, fresh bio-yoghurt beside them. Add a largish chunk of comb honey, take succulent bites out of the figs, and complement them with spoonfuls of yoghurt and honeycomb.

Per serving: *Calories 183 (From Fat 18); Fat 2 g (Saturated 1 g); Cholesterol 8 mg; Sodium 29 mg; Carbohydrate 39 g (Dietary Fibre 3 g); Protein 3 g.*

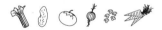

Melon with Mixed Berries

This is a dreamy breakfast to enjoy when you have plenty of time to consider the beneficial ingredients. All melon is delicious and health-giving, and with mixed berries it provides a delicious combination of fluid supply plus a powerful source of antioxidants. Use fresh blueberries from choice, or the frozen type if the fresh are unavailable.

Preparation time: *5 minutes*

Serves: *1*

½ charantais, honeydew or cantaloupe melon	*80–100 g mixture of fresh or frozen raspberries, strawberries, red or white currants*
1 handful fresh or frozen blueberries	*Honey*

(continued)

(continued)

1 Wash berries and top and tail the currants. Pat dry. Scrape out the seeds from the melon, place it on a plate and top/surround with your selection of berries and currants.

2 Drizzle with a little runny organic honey if you wish.

Per serving: Calories 314 (From Fat 7); Fat 1 g (Saturated 0 g); Cholesterol 0 mg; Sodium 55 mg; Carbohydrate 85 g (Dietary Fibre 10 g); Protein 4 g.

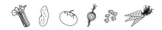

Really Delicious Porridge

Even if you've always hated porridge, this recipe may give you a pleasant surprise. I was amazed to discover that it really can be delicious. It also offers all the nerve-soothing properties of oats, and can help to keep you calm and focused for the rest of your day.

Preparation time: *10 minutes*

Serves: *1*

½ cup porridge oats

1 cup water

1 heaped tablespoon raisins, sultanas or currants

1 heaped tablespoon thick bio-yoghurt

1 Place oats and water in a saucepan and heat slowly, stirring, until rich and creamy, or place them in a microwaveable bowl or jug and cook for 2–3 minutes, depending on your oven. To remain true to the Scottish tradition, add a tiny pinch of salt.

2 Pour into a breakfast plate and stir in the dried fruit – during the 5–6 minutes required cooling time, they plump out and add a delicious sweetness to your cereal. Serve with the thick bio-yoghurt on top (for non-detoxers, substitute 1 tablespoon of double cream, and remind yourself of the cholesterol-lowering power of oats).

Per serving: Calories 190 (From Fat 32); Fat 4 g (Saturated 1 g); Cholesterol 2 mg; Sodium 11 mg; Carbohydrate 36 g (Dietary Fibre 4 g); Protein 6 g.

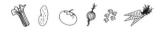

Chapter 14

Detox Soups

*M*ost people like soup, in one form or another. It's dead easy to eat, provides comfort and nourishment, and can be easily transported in a flask whenever you wish. Perhaps most of your experience of soup to date, has been of the tinned or packeted variety. Far from being a slog, many soups can be made in a matter of minutes, and can be made in larger than portion quantities and conveniently frozen.

Swimming in Soups

You *can* enjoy slightly richer 'cream' soups if you wish, adding low fat yoghurt or crème fraiche, but the simpler variety will probably appeal to you more during the early part of your detox, when your stomach and gut are cleansing themselves of excess fat and other toxins.

Stocking up on bouillon

Bouillon is basically the same as fish or meat stock minus the animal protein. I advise cutting corners unless you have all the time in the world, and use one of the powdered or cube varieties. You want a bouillon made from fresh and natural ingredients *only*, without a hint of preservative, colouring matter or other E-number items.

If you do decide to make it yourself, you can freeze any surplus, using the ice cube container. You can then shake the frozen cubes into a freezer bag, and use when you wish.

Your bouillon has *no* fixed quantities – make it a product of your creative imagination! Just heat a little olive oil (say 1–2 teaspoonfuls), and use it to soften as many peeled and chopped garlic cloves and medium-sized onions as you fancy. (Put the lid on and the small quantity of oil is compensated for by the condensed steam, which helps to cook the veg.)

When they're soft, throw in a couple of medium carrots, cut small, a couple of chopped celery stalks, a deseeded and sliced pepper of any colour, and a handful or two of any other veg you fancy.

Season with a little pepper (and tiny soupcon of salt), pour on 1 – 1.5 pints (800 – 1200 millilitres) boiling water, cover and simmer for 20 to 30 minutes. Put your feet up while the delicious smells of homemade bouillon waft enticingly around you.

Add a few chicken bones, the carcass or one or two wing joints or drumsticks for chicken bouillon – the chicken should be organic so that you can enjoy the full benefits of fresh poultry free from hormones, toxic feed residue and other nasties.

Living with the benefits

Not only will you be living with the detox benefits of the soup recipes and others in this book – you can also expect to experience increased energy, vitality and sense of well-being. The soups, in particular, enhance the cleansing and balancing (as well as reinvigorating) effects of detox, for two main reasons.

Firstly they supply extra liquid to encourage your kidneys and bowels to take a spring-clean (whatever the season of the year!).

Secondly, being very rich in antioxidants and other beneficial plant chemicals, they strengthen your immune defence system in its battle against released toxins and free radicals. Strengtening the immune system is absolutely central to detoxing, and it is rewarding to know that so much can be achieved through a few minutes' preparation and the eating or drinking of delicious foods. For details of the benefits of many of the ingredients in these recipes take a look back at Chapter 5.

Spring Vegetable Soup

This soup can surely put a spring in your step! While detoxing, you will be more aware of the need for cleansing. Your body is doing its best to purify itself, but you probably also want to see and feel fresh, natural, clean things around and inside you. Nothing fits the bill better than Spring greens or cabbage heart, flavourful, moist, bright- green and alive with freshness, and brimming with vitamins, minerals, and free radical-fighting antioxidants.

Preparation time: *15 minutes*

Cooking time: *20–30 minutes*

Serves: *1–2 hungry people*

1 teaspoon extra virgin olive oil

Bunch of spring onions or 1 large onion, finely chopped

2 fresh garlic cloves, chopped

1–2 handfuls spring greens or cabbage heart, roughly chopped

3 large tomatoes, chopped

1 tablespoon tomato puree

1 teaspoon marigold vegetable bouillon powder

0.6 litres (1 pint) of boiling water

1 Soften the onions and garlic in the olive oil, in a covered pan over a gentle heat.

2 Stir in the greens or cabbage, add 3–4 tablespoons water, cover and cook till leaves start to wilt.

3 Stir in the chopped tomatoes and their juice, the tomato puree, bouillon powder, and around 0.85 litres (1½ pint) of boiling water.

4 Continue cooking for 5–10 minutes, and season to taste with black pepper.

Per serving: *Calories 239 (From Fat 63); Fat 7 g (Saturated 1 g); Cholesterol 0 mg; Sodium 1,074 mg; Carbohydrate 44 g (Dietary Fibre 12 g); Protein 9 g. based on 1 serving.*

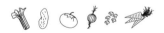

Spicy Parsnip Soup

Many British springs are wet and cold, and what could be nicer on a dank evening than warming, naturally sweet, and filling parsnip soup? Garlic is a great purifier of the blood and naturally lowers cholesterol (a common toxin!) Onions combat viral and bacterial infections, working alongside your bossy immune defence system; and turmeric turns off toxins linked to cancer triggers.

Special tool: *Blender or food processor*

Preparation time: *15–20 minutes*

Cooking time: *20–30 minutes*

Serves: *1*

1 teaspoon extra virgin olive oil

1 large onion, peeled and chopped

1 garlic clove, peeled and chopped

½ teaspoon ground turmeric

½ teaspoon curry powder

1 large or 2 medium parsnips, peeled and chopped

0.6–0.8 litres (1 to 1½ pints) boiling water or organic chicken stock

1 heaped tablespoon thick plain bio-yoghurt

Handful fresh parsley, chopped

1 Soften the garlic and onions in the olive oil over a medium heat, in covered pan.

2 Add spices, cook for 2–3 minutes, then add chopped parsnip. Stir to coat with the oil, then add the boiling water or organic chicken stock.

3 Return to the boil, turn down heat and simmer until soft (approx 10–15 minutes, depending on age of parsnips).

4 Remove from heat, allow to cool for a minute or two, then stir in the yoghurt.

5 Blend in 3 or 4 equal batches (to avoid splashing.) Serve at once, decorated with freshly chopped parsley.

Per serving: *Calories 257 (From Fat 51); Fat 6 g (Saturated 1 g); Cholesterol 1 mg; Sodium 420 mg; Carbohydrate 50 g (Dietary Fibre 10 g); Protein 6 g. Based on 1 serving.*

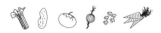

Chicken Consommé with Green Pepper Julienne

You need to keep your spirits up while detoxing, the first few hours or days of which can make some people tired and low. Fresh organic chicken is rich in the amino acid tryptophan used by the brain to manufacture a chemical called serotonin. This substance is directly related to mood, sleep, pain perception, and anxiety levels – we need serotonin in plentiful supply to keep the above functions ticking over normally. Some first-time detoxers also feel a bit anxious – and may sleep less well than usual as the cleansing stage of detox gets underway. High time to bring on the chicken consommé – with green pepper strips for added antioxidants!

Preparation time: *20–25 minutes*

Cooking time: *20 minutes + 1 hour*

Serves: *2–3*

1 cooked or uncooked organic chicken carcass	2 or 3 fresh bay leaves or ½ teaspoon dried herbs
1 onion, roughly chopped	Salt and pepper
1 carrot, roughly chopped	0.8–1.3 litres (1½ to 2 pints) cold water
3–4 cloves garlic, peeled and chopped	½ large green pepper, cut into julienne strips, for serving

1 Remove any fatty-looking appendages and skin from the carcass that may have been overlooked first time round. Leave a few scraps of meat on the bones to provide maximum flavour.

2 Place carcass in a large saucepan with the onion, carrot, garlic, and bay leaves, season with the salt and pepper, cover with the cold water, and bring to the boil.

3 Skim off any scum with a spoon, reduce the heat, partly cover, and simmer for approximately 1 hour, topping up liquid level as necessary (you want to end up with about 0.6 litres (1 pint) of liquid).

4 Strain the broth, removing all bones. You can leave in a little meat and vegetable fragments if you wish.

5 Cool to room temperature and place in fridge to set.

6 Before serving, blanch julienned green pepper strips in boiling water for 15 seconds, refresh under cold water, dry on kitchen paper, and use to decorate jellied consommé.

Per serving: Calories 50 (From Fat 16); Fat 2 g (Saturated 1 g); Cholesterol 12 mg; Sodium 160 mg; Carbohydrate 4 g (Dietary Fibre 1 g); Protein 5 g. Based on 2 servings.

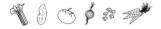

Simplest Detox Soup

You're on your lunch hour, you're very hungry and there's nothing detox-related in the fridge. You can sit down to a bowl of this delicious, filling soup in just minutes.

Special tool: Blender or food processor

Preparation time: *10–12 minutes*

Cooking time: *20–30 minutes*

Serves: *1–2*

2 teaspoons olive oil

½ to 1 teaspoon cumin seeds
(or ½ teaspoon ground spice)

1 medium onion, thinly sliced (used frozen ready-prepared, if desired)

1 or 2 celery stalks, washed and chopped

100 grams (4 ounces) red lentils

0.6–0.8 litres 1 to 1(½ pint) hot water or organic chicken or vegetable stock

1 Quickly heat the oil in a medium saucepan. Add the cumin seeds, stir to coat with the oil, then cook over a medium heat for 2–3 minutes.

2 Tip in the onion and celery, stir, and cook for another 4–5 minutes.

3 Tip in the lentils, stir once more, and add the hot water or stock.

4 Return to the boil, then reduce heat and simmer for 15–20 minutes.

5 Remove from heat, cool for a couple of minutes then whiz in the blender in 3 or 4 portions to avoid spillage. Heat again if required, serve, and enjoy.

Per serving: *Calories 449 (From Fat 84); Fat 9 g (Saturated 1 g); Cholesterol 0 mg; Sodium 87 mg; Carbohydrate 68 g (Dietary Fibre 18 g); Protein 26 g. based on 1 serving.*

Magic Mushroom and Fennel Soup

I don't mean the magic mushrooms that give you wonderful (or appalling) hallucinations, but a soup combining the supreme flavour of field mushrooms with fennel in a great detox soup.

Special tool: *Blender or food processor*

Preparation time: *10 minutes*

Cooking time: *35 minutes*

Serves: *2–3*

2 teaspoons olive oil

1 large onion, finely sliced

1 small fennel bulb, finely sliced

300 grams (12 ounces) large capped or field mushrooms, wiped, trimmed, and roughly chopped

0.7–1 litres (1¼ to 134 pints) organic chicken or vegetable stock

Salt and pepper

2 tablespoon fresh goat's or cow's bio-yoghurt

1 Heat olive oil in a medium-sized saucepan. Add the sliced onion, cook for a couple of minutes over a medium heat, then add the sliced fennel. Stir well, cover, and cook for 5–6 minutes.

2 Add the mushrooms, salt and pepper, and pour in the stock. Bring to the boil then reduce the heat and simmer for 25–30 minutes.

3 Remove from heat, allow it to cool for 2–3 minutes, then blitz it in a blender or food processor in 3 or 4 portions.

4 Return to saucepan, heat gently, and stir in the yoghurt. Serve, together with a slice or two of toasted wholemeal or sourdough bread.

Per serving: *Calories 146 (From Fat 60); Fat 7 g (Saturated 2 g); Cholesterol 0 mg; Sodium 720 mg; Carbohydrate 18 g (Dietary Fibre 4 g); Protein 6 g. based on 2 servings*

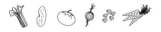

Tomato, Orange, and Ginger Soup

With tomato, orange, and ginger, this soup has a cleansing, astringent flavour as well as action. Tomato and orange supply natural vitamin C to boost your immune cells, and ginger soothes your digestive tract which *may* be feeling a little 'otherwise' when cleansing first starts (just take it easy, and remember to drink *lots* of water). In particular, ginger's anti-nausea action quells any queasiness you may experience, and encourage the release of mucus from your gut and nasal cavities.

Preparation time: 15–20 minutes

Cooking time: 25–30 minutes

Serves: 1–2

2 teaspoons olive oil

1 bunch spring onions, trimmed and chopped

300 grams (1 pound) fresh tomatoes, chopped

1 large orange

1.25 centimetres (½ inch) fresh ginger root, grated

0.6–0.8 litres (1 to 1½ pints) organic chicken or vegetable stock

Salt and pepper

1 Heat the oil and add the chopped spring onions and chopped tomatoes. Cook over a medium heat for 3 minutes.

2 Grate the orange peel and squeeze its juice. Add the grated peel and the squeezed juice to the saucepan.

3 Peel the segment of ginger, grate it, and put it aside. Cook the vegetables for 3 minutes, then add the grated ginger root.

4 Pour in the chicken or vegetable stock, season with pepper and salt. Bring to the boil, reduce heat, and simmer for 25 minutes. Serve as is, or blitz in a blender, and serve with a slice of wholemeal toast.

Per serving: *Calories 143 (From Fat 82); Fat 9 g (Saturated 2 g); Cholesterol 5 mg; Sodium 1,167 mg; Carbohydrate 15 g (Dietary Fibre 4 g); Protein 3 g. based on 2 servings.*

Galvanising Garlic Soup

This soup really *does* galvanise your immune system into action. It also reinvigorates your liver and eases colds, sore throats, and thick catarrh that interferes with normal breathing. It's a warming and delicious soup – provided you like garlic.

Special tool: *Blender or food processor*

Preparation time: *10 minutes*

Cooking time: *1 hour + 7–8 minutes*

Serves: *3–4*

1 whole head of garlic	*1 medium onion, finely sliced*
5–6 cups chicken broth	*Salt and pepper*
2–3 teaspoons olive oil	*Handful of fresh parsley, chopped*

1 Separate the garlic into cloves and place, unpeeled, in a saucepan with the broth. Heat until close to boiling, then reduce heat, cover tightly, and simmer for one hour.

2 Strain broth into another saucepan and remove the garlic from the skins when cool enough (a gentle squeeze at one end releases the deliciously squashy contents). Pop them straight into the blender.

3 Soften the onion in the olive oil for about 7 minutes, season to taste with salt and pepper, and place in a blender together with the garlic and 2 cups of the broth. Process until smooth and then combine with remaining broth. Reheat gently and serve scattered with chopped parsley.

Per serving: *Calories 120 (From Fat 88); Fat 10 g (Saturated 2 g); Cholesterol 8 mg; Sodium 1,767 mg; Carbohydrate 6 g (Dietary Fibre 1 g); Protein 3 g.*

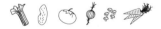

Clear Soup with Tofu and Wakame

Delicious and nourishing, this Japanese soup is perfect for serving dinner guests if you find yourself entertaining during a detox. It uses *dashi* – a basic stock used in nearly all Japanese dishes. The most common form is made from dried kelp, water, and flakes of dried bonito (fish.) You can also buy instant dashi as a concentrated liquid or as granules that you dilute with water according to your personal taste or the recipe concerned.

This recipe also calls for *shoyu,* Japanese soy sauce, which is milder and less salty than the Chinese variety (although you can use the latter in moderation, in an emergency.) Choose one of the better quality soy sauces, free from all artificial additives, especially monosodium glutamate (MSG). Try Japanese food Web sites and Asian grocers to find these products.

Special tool: *Small flower-shaped cutter (optional).*

Preparation time: *10–20 minutes*

Cooking time: *5–6 minutes*

Serves: *4*

5 grams dried wakame (seaweed)

200 grams (8 ounces) firm tofu, cut into 8 slices.

4 cups (1 litre) dashi

1 tablespoon sake (dry rice wine) or dry sherry

2 teaspoons light Japanese soy sauce (shoyu)

1 teaspoon finely shredded lemon peel

1 Ensure that the tofu is at room temperature.

2 Place seaweed in a small bowl, cover with cold water, and leave to soften (about 10 minutes). Drain it, squeeze out excess water, and chop coarsely, removing any tough ribs.

3 Meanwhile, cut a flower shape from each of the tofu slices using a 3.5-centimetre (1⅛ in) cutter (you will probably find this size if you decide to buy a flower-shaped cutter). Alternatively, cut fancy shapes yourself using a small, sharp knife, or simply chop tofu into 1.25-centimetre (½ inch) cubes.

4 Divide seaweed and tofu among four serving bowls. Heat the dashi to boiling point in a medium saucepan, stir in sake (or sherry) and soy sauce. Divide soup among the serving bowls and sprinkle with lemon peel.

Per serving: Calories 42 (From Fat 13); Fat 1 g (Saturated 0 g); Cholesterol 0 mg; Sodium 2,314 mg; Carbohydrate 2 g (Dietary Fibre 0 g); Protein 4 g.

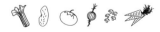

Essential Celery Soup

Celery soup is a great source of comfort when you're cold, empty, and too tired to cook. In this recipe, the celery seeds enhance the essential flavour of the celery without having to fry the vegetables first.

Preparation time: *10 minutes*

Cooking time: *1 hour or a bit less*

Serves: *3–4*

1 head of celery, trimmed and chopped into bite-size pieces (save one or two stalks or the knobbly bit at the base for serving)

1 medium onion, peeled and sliced

1.1 litres (2 pints) organic chicken or vegetable stock or bouillon

Salt and pepper

1 heaped teaspoon celery seeds

Goat's or cow's bio-yoghurt or low fat fromage frais, to serve

1 Place celery and onion in a large saucepan with the stock, bring briefly to the boil, then simmer, partly covered, for about 45 minutes until very soft.

2 Return to the pan, season, add the celery seeds, and heat thoroughly for 5–10 minutes. Pour it in small quantities depending on the size of your blender, and, when pureed, sieve it and pour it into serving bowl with 1 dessertspoon of yoghurt or fromage frais floating on the surface, with an extra sprinkle of celery seeds on top. Serve with a crunchy stalk or two and/or pieces of the root.

Remember the soup may be very hot – blend in small quantities to avoid overspill and possible scalding.

Vary It! *Omit the sieving and/or blending if you wish. This soup is equally delicious if you leave the vegetables just as they are.*

Per serving: *Calories 77 (From Fat 8); Fat 1 g (Saturated 0 g); Cholesterol 0 mg; Sodium 912 mg; Carbohydrate 17 g (Dietary Fibre 6 g); Protein 4 g.*

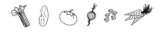

Mediterranean Tomato Soup

This wonderful detox soup provides omega-3 fatty acids (in the olive oil) and is rich in antioxidants, especially the cancer-combating lycopene (cooking the tomatoes enhances the availability of lycopene).

 To peel tomatoes easily, drop them into boiling water for one minute, then dip them in cold water. Peel off the skin when the tomatoes are cool enough to handle.

Preparation time: *15 minutes*

Cooking time: *30–40 minutes*

Serves: *2–3*

2 tablespoons olive oil

1 medium leek, sliced

2 carrots, finely diced

2 celery stalks

2 to 3 cloves of garlic, peeled and crushed

1.5 kilograms (3 pounds) ripe tomatoes, peeled and chopped

½ cup chopped fresh basil or ½ teaspoon dried basil

1 level teaspoon of soft brown sugar

Salt and pepper

1 Heat the oil in a large saucepan, then add the leek, carrots, celery and garlic, and cook gently until tender (15 to 20 mins over a medium to low heat). Meanwhile, skin the tomatoes by dropping them into boiling water for 1 minute, refreshing in cold water, and peeling off the skin when cool enough to handle. Chop the tomatoes.

2 Add the tomatoes, together with the basil and sugar, to the softened vegetables. Season with salt and pepper to taste, cover and simmer gently for 30 minutes.

Per serving: *Calories 132 (From Fat 31); Fat 4 g (Saturated 1 g); Cholesterol 0 mg; Sodium 225 mg; Carbohydrate 25 g (Dietary Fibre 6 g); Protein 4 g.*

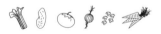

Chapter 15

Detox Salads

*A*re you detoxing for the first time? Or simply reading this book out of interest? Whatever your ideas on the subject, the word 'salads' must surely figure in huge capitals in your mind's eye. Perhaps you've imagined days spent eating the same boring old lettuce, tomatoes, and cucumber – albeit with a nod to modern eating with the addition of a few raddiccio leaves (for instance), or a handful of chopped fresh herbs.

Not the most alluring of gustatory prospects, but, detox is soooo valuable, surely it's worth suffering for? Well, no. Salads can be valuable detox fodder without being in the least off-putting – as a glance at the above recipe list shows you. While the emphasis remains upon fresh vegetables and fruit, low fat, easily-digested protein also figures in the form of seafood and chicken. So there should, hopefully, be something here for everyone.

A Salad a Day Keeps the Toxins at Bay!

Refreshment comes from cool, moist, juicy foods with a high water content – all of which combat dehydration and encourage the skin and kidneys to eliminate water-soluble toxins. And the fresh veg and fruit that supply the basis of these salads encourage toxin elimination and combat their damaging effects by strengthening your immune defence system. Pressed or squeezed juices, salad leaves, raw or lightly cooked vegetables, and fruit are good choices. You also need lean protein or complex carbohydrate to satisfy hunger pangs and restore your energy.

Lunch hour? Time for refreshment!

You can snack on salad foods whenever you want, but I'm assuming here that you eat your daily salad at lunchtime. You may have less time to prepare food in the middle of the day or perhaps you take a packed lunch in to work or school. Salads tend to be highly portable, can be prepared the night before, and are ready to go next day, cool and fresh from the refrigerator.

Breakfast is sometimes referred to as the most essential meal of the day, but I believe that all meals are equally important – they just serve different purposes. When you're detoxing, you need to avoid both the low blood sugar levels linked to long gaps between meals, *and* the drowsiness and bloating that carbohydrate foods can cause.

Halfway through the day, you need sustenance that can refresh you after your morning's activities, replenish your energy, and top up your *antioxidants* (nutrients that combat the ill effects of *free radicals,* hyperactive oxygen molecules produced throughout your body and linked to cancer, ageing, and allergic illnesses.)

 Everyone needs antioxidants, especially city dwellers and those travelling or working in crowded conditions. Antioxidants help to protect the whole body from free radical damage. You have a particularly pressing need of antioxidants when you're detoxing in order to fight free radicals and to help your liver, lungs, kidneys, skin, and bowel neutralise and eliminate accumulated toxins.

To read about the benefits of many of the ingredients in the recipes take a look back at Chapter 5.

Side-stepping unhealthy ingredients

Salads are brimful of antioxidants and are excellent for detoxing – as you already know. But you can undo all a salad's benefits by including unsuitable ingredients. The following sections cover the chief items you need to avoid.

Forgoing unhealthy fats

Trans-fatty acids have an anti-vitamin effect in the body and counteract the benefits of free radicals. They are formed when healthy
plant fats such as cis-linoleic acid are processed at high temperatures. The cheaper brands of cooking oil and butter substitutes
use this process. Only cold-pressed plant-food oils, such as extra
virgin olive and sunflower oils, contain nutrient fatty acids in their
healthy 'cis' forms.

Saturated animal fats may be easier to spot than trans-fats because
you are more aware of them. An organic egg added to a salad or
used to make mayonnaise can be a healthy addition while detoxing; but fatty meats such as cold roast pork, lamb, beef, or chicken
with its skin, demand extra work of the liver and gall bladder
which are working flat out to expel your toxin load. And butter
(including the so-called 'light' varieties) is out, because of the high
saturated fat content.

Subtracting additives

'Additives' are a collective name for artificial substance added to a
food, such as colourings, 'fillers', flavourings, and preservatives
most often found in commercial sauces and snack foods (such as
coloured or flavoured seeds, crisps, and their equivalents), tinned
meat and fish, and commercially prepared pies, flans, and tarts.

Even the most expensive brands of mayonnaise are unlikely to be
entirely additive-free, and few, if any, are made entirely from 100 per
cent guaranteed organic produce including extra virgin olive oil.

When detoxing, you are probably better off making your own mayonnaise, a recipe for which you can find later in this chapter.

Throwing over the salt

Salt is the last thing your kidneys need when labouring to expel
lots of toxins in your urine. Avoid sprinkling it on salad leaves and
veg, and steer clear of sauces and other condiments to which it
has been added.

Cutting down on carbohydrates

Go without that tempting roll or slice of bread you usually eat with
a salad. I am assuming your usual bread and rolls are white, and
the recipes in this section provide healthier alternatives to bulk
out your salad meal; alternatively, eat with a slice of organic sourdough or rye bread, a few butter beans, a sweet potato, steamed
till soft and sliced.

Boiled potatoes have a high glycaemic index (G.I.), meaning that they may boost your blood sugar levels too rapidly, thereby producing a high blood sugar level followed by a steep fall, leaving you shaky and weak. Avoid them while detoxing.

Detouring around dairy

You need dairy foods for their nutrient content, especially calcium. But their full-fat form is high in saturated fat, and you should use them sparingly while detoxing, making sure you avoid cheeses, and similar products unless they are low in saturated fat.

Salad Selections

Detox salads can contain a wide selection of delectable ingredients, some of which you will find in the following recipes. And if you like the general idea of a particular salad but not one of its ingredients (scallops, say, or watercress) let your imagination roam.... Stick to the fresh, low fat, natural, organic basis of detox eating and select a substitute that does appeal. White crab meat (for example) may suit you well, or rocket or baby spinach leaves instead of watercress or other leafy suggestions.

Asparagus and Blood Orange Salad

This is an excellent detox salad to prepare for yourself if you fancy something out of the ordinary. And it's an equally good choice for a dinner party first course when something unusual, flavoursome, and visually enticing is the order of the day. (Plus, it demands minimum hoo-hah in the kitchen!)

Preparation time: _20–30 minutes_

Cooking time: _4–7 minutes (the older and fatter the asparagus, the longer it takes to soften)_

Serves: _1_

6–12 fresh asparagus spears (depending on size)

For mayonnaise:

1 organic egg yolk

Juice of 1 organic blood orange

½ teaspoon Dijon mustard

0.06 litre (2 fluid ounces) olive oil

1 Peel white asparagus; leave green as it is. Trim off stalk ends. Steam according to the times suggested above. Then refresh the asparagus in cold water.

2 Meanwhile (or beforehand), make the mayonnaise: whisk together the egg yolk, juice, and mustard, then add olive oil in a thin and steady stream, whisking constantly, until you have a glossy, thick emulsion. Stir in a little extra blood orange juice to taste.

Vary It! *An ordinary orange is just as good, but blood orange juice is prettier.*

Per serving: *Calories 231 (From Fat 173); Fat 19 g (Saturated 4 g); Cholesterol 213 mg; Sodium 81 mg; Carbohydrate 11 g (Dietary Fibre 2 g); Protein 6 g. Analysed with 1 tbsp olive oil.*

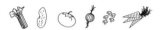

Fennel, Caper, and Parmesan Salad

This salad will appeal to you if you are already a fennel fan or simply like aniseed flavour.

Preparation time: *10–15 minutes*

Serves: *2–3*

For the salad:

1 small fennel bulb, trimmed and sliced into thin rounds

2–3 handfuls of watercress

1 heaped tablespoon capers

50–75 grams (2–3 ounces) Parmesan cheese, grated

For the dressing:

1 tablespoon organic balsamic vinegar

1 tablespoon extra virgin olive oil

Pinch of salt, freshly ground black pepper

1 Mix the first four ingredients together.

2 Whisk the vinegar, oil, salt, and pepper together until you achieve a fine emulsion. Use to dress the salad and toss the salad for an even distribution of dressing.

Vary It! *As an alternative to watercress, choose other strong-tasting salad leaves such as radiccio or rocket.*

Per serving: *Calories 234 (From Fat 140); Fat 16 g (Saturated 6 g); Cholesterol 22 mg; Sodium 793 mg; Carbohydrate 11 g (Dietary Fibre 4 g); Protein 14 g. Based on 2 servings.*

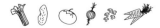

Almost Instant Warm Bean Shoot Salad

This takes no time to prepare. It's also low in calories, filling, warming, and rich in vitamins, minerals, and lycopene.

Preparation time: *5– 7 minutes*

Cooking time: *1–2 minutes or 5–7 minutes depending on cooking method*

Serves: *1 hungry person or 2 as a side dish*

175–200 grams (7–8 ounces) fresh bean shoots	Small tin bamboo shoots, drained and cut into slices
2–3 cloves garlic, peeled and chopped	2–3 tablespoons soy sauce or 1 heaped tablespoon tomato puree

1 Boil enough water to cover the ingredients in a saucepan and add the bean shoots and garlic, cooking them for 1½–2 minutes, or place the bean shoots and garlic in a sieve, cover with a saucepan lid and steam them over the boiling water for 5–6 minutes (or a bit longer if you like them on the soft side). Drain thoroughly.

2 Mix in the sliced bamboo shoots, to which add bulk, and the soy sauce or the tomato puree.

Per serving: Calories 138 (From Fat 13); Fat 1 g (Saturated 0 g); Cholesterol 0 mg; Sodium 1,871 mg; Carbohydrate 22 g (Dietary Fibre 7 g); Protein 15 g. Based on one serving.

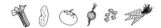

Spinach, Mung Bean, and Beetroot Salad

This is a most refreshing salad, best chilled for 2–3 hours before eating.

Preparation time: *10–15 mins*

Serves: *2–3, or 4 as a side salad*

For the salad:

100 grams (4 ounces) baby spinach leaves	Handful of sprouting mung beans
75 grams (3 ounces) alfalfa sprouts	3–4 small cooked beetroots, thickly sliced
2–3 carrots, finely sliced	

For the dressing:

1 tablespoon cider vinegar

1 dessertspoon runny honey

1 teaspoon orange juice

Snipped chives to taste

Salt and pepper

1 Whisk together the dressing ingredients.

2 Mix spinach, alfalfa sprouts, carrots, mung bean sprouts, and beetroot in a bowl, and toss in the dressing.

Tip: *The beetroot will bleed onto the other ingredients. If this worries you (there is no reason why it should nutritionally), add the beetroot chunks shortly before serving.*

Per serving: *Calories 132 (From Fat 5); Fat 1 g (Saturated 0 g); Cholesterol 0 mg; Sodium 339 mg; Carbohydrate 30 g (Dietary Fibre 8 g); Protein 7 g.*

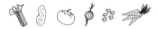

'Hot' Tuna Salad

This salad is hot in the spicy sense, but you can also serve it heated or luke-warm, if you prefer. It is good during detox to counteract too many bland foods.

Preparation time: *10 minutes*

Cooking time: *8–10 minutes depending on thickness of fish*

Serves: *4–6*

175– 200 grams (7–8 ounces) tuna, fresh or tinned in oil

150–200 grams (6–8 ounces) organic brown rice, cooked

20 radishes, thinly sliced

150 grams (6 ounces) green or runner beans, cooked

½ cucumber, thinly sliced

3–4 tablespoon Japanese shoyu or standard soy sauce

2½–5 centimetres (1–2 inches) fresh ginger root, peeled and grated

2 handfuls of nasturtium leaves or mustard and cress

2 handfuls nasturtium flowers

1 Steam or microwave fresh fish, or drain tinned tuna of its oil. Divide into largish flakes.

2 Mix the tuna gently into the cooked rice, together with the radishes, beans, cucumber, shoyu, and grated ginger root.

(continued)

(continued)

3 Just before serving, stir in the salad leaves or cress, and decorate the salad and its bowl with the nasturtium flowers, which are edible.

Tip: The quantities of radishes, shoyu, peppery leaves, and ginger are guide-lines only: vary according to taste.

Per serving: *Calories 275 (From Fat 32); Fat 4 g (Saturated 0 g); Cholesterol 30 mg; Sodium 1,966 mg; Carbohydrate 29 g (Dietary Fibre 6 g); Protein 33 g. Based on 2 servings.*

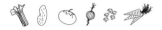

Traditional English Salad

This may come as a surprise, because a traditional English salad is a time-honoured cliché for the unattractive side of our eating habits. However, you may well be one of the many now growing their own veg; alternatively, fresh organic produce is now readily available throughout the year. You can't feel experimental and innovative every day.

Preparation time: *5 minutes*

Serves: *4–6*

For the salad:

I large English cos lettuce

4–5 vine tomatoes, depending on size, sliced

11–12 spring onions, sliced

1 medium beetroot, cooked, quartered

15-centimetre (6-inch) piece of cucumber thinly sliced.

Punnet of mustard and cress

15–20 radishes

For the dressing:

2 tablespoons fresh lemon juice

1 dessertspoon runny honey

1 tablespoon olive oil

Pinch of mixed herbs

Salt and pepper

1 Mix the lemon juice, honey, olive oil, and herbs together, and season with a grind of pepper and a pinch of salt.

2 Wash and trim the salad ingredients, shake well to remove excess water and, if necessary, pat dry with kitchen paper. Keep all ingredients in the fridge and assemble just before eating, slicing/chopping vegetables as you prefer. Serve the dressing separately.

Per serving: *Calories 94 (From Fat 8); Fat 1 g (Saturated 0 g); Cholesterol 0 mg; Sodium 222 mg; Carbohydrate 20 g (Dietary Fibre 6 g); Protein 5 g.*

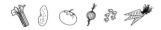

Nutty Lamb's Lettuce Salad with Sesame Dressing

This salad is a good choice if you feel at all deprived while detoxing, and yearn for something that tastes rich and decadent.

Special tool: Blender or food processor

Preparation time: 20 minutes

Cooking time: 2–3 mins for nuts, 4–5 mins for sweet corns depending upon size and heat applied.

Serves: 1–2

For the salad:

6–8 baby sweet corns

1 handful hazelnuts

2–3 handfuls lamb's lettuce

6–8 vine cherry tomatoes, halved

¼ medium Spanish onion, very thinly sliced

For the dressing:

Juice of 1 lime

2 tablespoons tahini (sesame seed paste)

1–2 tablespoons soy sauce to taste

1–2 tablespoons sesame oil to taste

1 garlic clove, finely chopped

1 Blend the dressing ingredients in a blender or food processor. Set aside.

2 Dry-fry the baby sweet corns in a frying pan over moderate heat. Heat a clean dry frying pan and place within it the baby sweet corn. Toss them around with a fork. When they are done, they are softish and perhaps slightly browned in places.

3. Roast the hazelnuts on a tray under a medium grill until light brown. Place the nuts on a clean grilling tray, and place under a medium to fairly hot grill, checking them every minute or so to avoid burning.

4 Assemble lamb's lettuce and halved cherry tomatoes in a glass dish, Add the baby sweet corns and hazelnuts. Toss in dressing just before eating, or serve dressing separately.

Tip: Don't worry if the sweet corns become slightly blackened while dry-frying; this only improves their flavour.

Tip: Any remaining dressing keeps well for 2–3 weeks in the fridge in a screw-top jar or bottle.

(continued)

(continued)

> ***Vary It!*** *If you love roast hazelnuts, substituting hazelnut butter and oil for the tahini and sesame oil elevates this eating experience to heavenly heights. Hazelnut butter is available at online Web sites (check Google) and in many good health food stores. If you cannot find hazelnut oil, use peanut or safflower oil instead.*

Per serving: *Calories 607 (From Fat 434); Fat 48 g (Saturated 6 g); Cholesterol 0 mg; Sodium 978 mg; Carbohydrate 38 g (Dietary Fibre 11g); Protein 16 g. Based on one serving.*

Scallop, Chicory, and Pomegranate Salad

This mixture of flavours works well; the slightly bitter chicory counterbalances the richness of the scallops, which contain most of the essential amino acids, especially methionine, and the good-mood-linked tryptophan and the pomegranate adds piquancy and beauty (plus tons of antioxidants!)

Preparation time: *20–30 minutes*

Cooking time: *15–20 minutes*

Serves: *1–2*

1 ripe pomegranate	*2–3 scallops*
1 head of chicory, separated into leaves	*Salt and pepper to taste*
Small bunch spring onions, washed and trimmed	*1 to 2 tablespoons olive oil*
	1 tablespoon fresh bread crumbs
15-centimetre (6-inch) piece of cucumber, peeled and chopped	*Several sprigs fresh parsley*

1 Halve the pomegranate and scoop out the seeds, avoiding the cream-coloured membrane. Save any juice, and place the seeds and flesh to one side.

2 Assemble the chicory leaves, spring onions, and cucumber in a dish.

3 Wipe scallops with a damp cloth and place them in a small baking dish. Season with salt and pepper, drizzle with olive oil and scatter over the bread crumbs and parsley. Cover, and bake in the centre of a moderate oven for 15–20 minutes; the scallops are done when the flesh is opaque, soft, and oozing delicious juices.

4 Combine scallops, the crumbs, and salad, dot liberally with pomegranate seeds, and dress the salad with a mixture of pan and pomegranate juices, a grind of salt and pepper, and a drizzle of olive oil.

Tip: *Try to find scallops complete with their bright orange roes, which perfectly complement the delicious white meat.*

Per serving: *Calories 363 (From Fat 151); Fat 17 g (Saturated 2 g); Cholesterol 20 mg; Sodium 499 mg; Carbohydrate 42 g (Dietary Fibre 6 g); Protein 15 g. Based on one serving.*

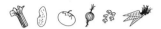

Couscous, Sun-dried Tomato, and Chicken Salad

This filling, satisfying salad does equally well as a lunch dish when you need to top up your energy levels or as a supper or dinner meal in the evening.

Preparation time: *20 minutes*

Cooking time: *15 minutes*

Serves: *1*

2 heaped tablespoon couscous	*1 chicken breast, finely sliced*
1½ tablespoons soy sauce	*4–5 sun-dried tomatoes, preserved in oil*
1–2 dessertspoons of oil from sun-dried tomatoes	*Handful of watercress or baby spinach leaves*
3–4 cloves of garlic, crushed	*Handful of walnuts, chopped*

1 Place couscous in a jug or basin and pour over just enough boiling water to thoroughly coat the grains. Mix thoroughly. When the couscous is fully hydrated (swollen), stir in the soy sauce and set it aside.

2 Heat 1 dessertspoon of sun-dried tomato oil in a frying-pan, and cook garlic until soft. Remove garlic and set aside, add a drop more oil and fry the sliced chicken breast until it's cooked through, which takes about 7 minutes over a medium heat. Add the sun-dried tomatoes 3–4 minutes before the chicken is fully cooked.

3 To assemble the salad, add the couscous to the chicken pan, together with the garlic and watercress or spinach leaves. Heat gently, stirring, until the leaves wilt. Serve, scattered with the chopped walnuts.

Per serving: *Calories 323 (From Fat 132); Fat 15 g (Saturated 2 g); Cholesterol 73 mg; Sodium 1,485 mg; Carbohydrate 14 g (Dietary Fibre 2 g); Protein 35 g.*

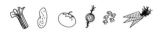

Arabian Nights Salad

Pleasant and easy to eat, this salad is good with vegetable, chicken, or fish kebabs, or with sliced lamb's liver, cooked very gently in a little olive oil.

Preparation time: *5 minutes plus chilling time*

Serves: *2*

2–3 large oranges (use blood oranges if possible)

1 dessertspoon rosewater

1 dessertspoon mineral water

2 dozen or so black olives

1 large leek, washed and finely sliced

Small handful of fresh tarragon leaves, crushed or ½ teaspoon dried tarragon

Salt and pepper to taste

1 Peel oranges, remove every scrap of pith, and slice thinly into a bowl, catching all the juice. Mix the rosewater with an equal volume of mineral water, and pour over fruit.

2 Stone the olives if you like and combine them with the oranges and sliced leek.

3 Chill well, and stir in the tarragon, salt and pepper a couple of hours before serving.

Tip: *Use only the white portion of the leek, after sluicing well between the layers to remove grit and cutting off the end root.*

Per serving: *Calories 242 (From Fat 92); Fat 10 g (Saturated 0 g); Cholesterol 0 mg; Sodium 595 mg; Carbohydrate 37 g (Dietary Fibre 6 g); Protein 2 g.*

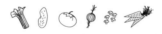

Chapter 16

Detox Snacks, Dips, and Spreads

In This Chapter

▶ Making a good choice of dip and spread ingredients

▶ Preparing dip and spread recipes

*T*he last thing you want to feel when detoxing or, indeed, during any kind of diet, is deprived. You need to make the experience a pleasant one. And if you don't enjoy your detox regimen, you may well not complete the number of days you had planned and you're even less likely to repeat the experience. In this chapter, I offer recipes that offer tasty treats that make you feel pampered instead of deprived.

Spreading the Treats

When you change your ordinary eating pattern for a detox diet you eliminate the artificial additives, high fat, and high sugar present in most processed and convenience foods. As a result you're likely to enjoy 'good plain food' more than you did previously because you become more aware of its taste and texture. Your enjoyment, however, won't prevent you from secretly longing for some sort of food indulgence, be it sweet, rich, or just plain luxurious. The craving is even stronger if you tend to *comfort eat,* turning to food in moments of emotional need.

Cravings for, and comfort-eating, foods high in fat, sugar, and so on, can often be brought to heel with the use of cunning substitutes. Let's suppose, for example, that you are pining for Welsh rarebit on toast, crumpets oozing with melted butter, or a plate of strawberries piled with sugar and whipped cream.

While keeping down the overall fat and sugar content, it's perfectly possible to use cold-pressed vegetable oils and naturally sweet fruit products (such as organic apple or pear spread) in sufficient amounts to make a dip, spread, or sweet treat rich and satisfying to your taste buds. And this can be achieved using detox foods without threatening your overall fat intake – or bumping up the calories if calories matter especially to you. Examples of snacks which combine pleasure with high nutritional intake while boosting toxin elimination include guacamole, which uses mashed ripe avocado, hummus which utilises sesame seed paste (tahini), and smoked mackerel pâté.

You can also make a pleasantly creamy topping for fresh fruit (for instance) using yoghurt and a little naturally sweet juice from a fresh paw paw, mango, or similar fruit.

Finding detoxing snacks

When detoxing, don't you just *long* for delicious crisps, corn chips, and chunks of supermarket focaccio to scoop up rich, dreamy dips and spreads? Well, there's no need to, if you box clever – you *can* have your cake and eat it in this instance, and score top detox marks while dipping and spreading to your heart's content.

Here are a few suggestions:

Crudités

Pre-detox, you may have considered crudites 'just boring raw vegetables', but experiment with a few you haven't tried for scooping up healthy dips. Spring onions, small segments of the tender inner segments of a fresh leek, newly washed young carrots, strips of courgette, florets of broccoli or cauliflower, and cucumber or sweet pepper rings are all excellent choices.

Or, if you want a new experience, try grapes, strawberries, slices of a firm pear or an apple, if you like sweet and sour flavour combinations (always a very popular choice when eating Chinese food). You may like the partnership of apple with hummous (for example), orange slices and tzatziki, or cherries and tapenade.

Bread dippers

If you buy an organic, wholegrain loaf, toast slices, cut into small triangles and use for dipping.

Equally healthy choices include a poppadom baked hard in the oven for a few minutes, and torn into 'dipable' pieces.

Alternatively, look for additive-free breadsticks from supermarkets and health shops. Sourdough, corn and rye breads are very wholesome and aid aspects of detox (nutrient supply, encourage release of bowel toxins) and I do urge you to try Pumpernickel (Westphalian rye bread) – heavy, moist, filling, delectable with sweet and sour dips alike.

Dried vegetables and fruit

All the crisps I have seen are pretty high in fat (and potatoes themselves have a high-G.I. rating). You can buy dehydrator kitchen appliances which dry-slice fruit and vegetables, ideal (perfect, in fact!) for dipping and snacking detox purposes. They tend to be pricey (£74 is the cheapest I have found on the Internet) so my best advice is to purchase *Making and Using Dried Fruits* by Phyllis Hobson (Storey Books), available on the www.Amazon.co.uk Web site for £7.25 (paperback edition). It has a ***** rating.

Making sure your snacks aren't bad

Foods to avoid when choosing different spread ingredients on a detox regimen include high-fat dairy products such as full-fat crème fraiche, full-fat yoghurt, full-fat cheeses, and commercial and full-fat mayonnaise. Stay away from fattening snacks like pork scratchings and butter or margarine containing hydrogenated vegetable oil.

Others to avoid are the foods you may have chosen in the past to use for dipping and spreading. Low G.I. carbohydrates such as white bread and potato slices are typical (if slightly healthier) examples, while the worst you can choose are the high-fat, high-chemical additive and usually high-salt, high-sugar types of 'handy snacks' so freely available at supermarket check-outs and sweet shops.

Can butter contain hydrogenated vegetable oil? Not 'whole' butter, but the 'light' sort with fewer fat calories can be a mixture of true butter with its saturated fats, plus hydrogenated vegetable oils.

Dishing Up Dips and Spreads

The object throughout the following dips and spreads, is to encourage you to choose something extra delicious once or twice a day.

Guacamole

Guacamole is a delicious and satisfying dip for eating with organic oat cakes, organic Pumpernickel (Westphalia rye bread), or even as a single spoonful on its own, when your day proves long and hard.

Corn chips *are* out of bounds if (as is true of all the brands I have researched) – they contain hydrogenated vegetable oils and/or saturated fats in their preparation.

Preparation time: *15 minutes*

Serves: *1–2*

1 large ripe avocado	*Juice of half a lemon, or 1 to*
2 tablespoons of reduced-fat plain Greek yoghurt	*2 tablespoons soy sauce*
	½ teaspoon of dried chilli flakes
	Sea salt and freshly ground black pepper

1 Halve the avocado lengthways, slide the halves apart, and discard the central stone. Cut each half in half again, down its length; then simply peel the skin off the four quarters. Check inside the skins before discarding them for any remaining bright green flesh, since this is often the most succulent.

2 Mash the avocado thoroughly using a fork, then stir in the yoghurt and mix thoroughly.

3 Now add the lemon juice (or soy sauce) stirring well. Stir in the dried chilli flakes and season lightly with freshly ground black pepper and a little sea salt to taste. Your dip is now ready, so dive in!

Per serving: *Calories 367 (From Fat 295); Fat 33 g (Saturated 6 g); Cholesterol 4 mg; Sodium 1,246 mg; Carbohydrate 17 g (Dietary Fibre 11 g); Protein 8 g. Based on 1 serving.*

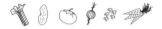

Hummus

Nutty and succulent, the sesame seed paste makes hummus taste sinfully indulgent, but the fibre content encourages the bowel to eliminate toxins and other waste, and the omega-6 fatty acids boost your immune system's ability to shake off toxins.

Speciality tools: *Blender*

Preparation time: *15 minutes*

Serves: *2–3*

150-gram (5-ounce) tin of organic chick-peas

1 tablespoon extra virgin olive oil

1 tablespoon sesame oil

Grated zest and squeezed juice of 1 large lemon

3 garlic cloves, crushed

75 grams (3 ounces) organic tahini sesame paste

Chopped fresh parsley for garnish

A pinch of sea salt and freshly ground black pepper.

1 Drain the chick-peas, saving the liquid, and place them in a blender or food processor with the oils, lemon juice, zest, and garlic.

2 Add about half the liquid from the tin, blend until the mixture looks like pale peanut butter, then add the tahini paste. Blend again. If the blender clogs, add a little more liquid. Season to taste and garnish with the parsley.

Per serving: Calories 382 (From Fat 290); Fat 32 g (Saturated 4 g); Cholesterol 0 mg; Sodium 234 mg; Carbohydrate 20 g (Dietary Fibre 6 g); Protein 10 g. Based on 2 servings.

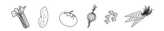

Tzatziki

This Greek cucumber dish is very refreshing when temperatures soar, and an equally pleasant accompaniment to hot, spicy food in cold weather. Tzatziki is rich in antioxidants such as chlorophyll and vitamin C for fighting free radicals (the hyperactive oxygen molecules that damage tissue), as well as calcium for calm nerves and strong bones and teeth.

Preparation time: *10 minutes*

Serves: *4*

Half a large cucumber

10 tablespoons (150 mls) reduced fat plain yoghurt

3 to 4 spring onions, trimmed and chopped finely

2 garlic cloves, crushed

1 tablespoon fresh mint

1 Rinse the cucumber, pat dry, trim off the end, and chop to bite-size pieces.

2 Mix the cucumber pieces into the yoghurt together with the garlic, spring onions, and fresh mint. When they are really amalgamated, bind together and chill for at least an hour before serving.

Per serving: Calories 74 (From Fat 10); Fat 1 g (Saturated 1 g); Cholesterol 6 mg; Sodium 75 mg; Carbohydrate 11 g (Dietary Fibre 1 g); Protein 6 g.

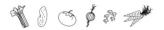

Bean and Walnut Dip

This dish is perfect as a starter course or as a main course with lots of fresh vegetable crudités to dip in.

Specialty tools: *Food processor or blender*

Preparation time: *15 minutes*

Serves: *3–4*

310-gram (10-ounce) can of organic butter beans, or red kidney beans, drained and rinsed

1 tablespoon organic cold-pressed olive oil

2 garlic cloves, crushed

1 tablespoon tomato purée (optional)

Sea salt and freshly ground black pepper

2 tablespoons walnut halves, in small pieces

2 tablespoons chopped mixed fresh herbs, such as mint, parsley, chives

1 Process the beans, oil, garlic, and tomato purée (if desired) in a food processor or blender until smooth.

2 Place in dish, season lightly with salt and pepper, and stir in the walnut pieces and herbs. Serve with oatcakes, small wedges of toasted organic pitta bread, or freshly chopped celery stalks.

Per serving: *Calories 124 (From Fat 65); Fat 7 g (Saturated 1 g); Cholesterol 0 mg; Sodium 394 mg; Carbohydrate 15 g (Dietary Fibre 4 g); Protein 5 g. Based on 3 servings.*

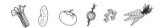

Aubergine and Hazelnut Dip

This is rich in flavour and texture as well as in vitamin C, omega-6 oils, and bio-flavonoids, among other nutrients.

Specialty tools: *Blender, sieve*

Preparation time: *20 minutes*

Cooking time: *35–45 minutes*

Serves: *6–8*

2 large aubergines, about 850 grams (2 pounds) in weight

2 garlic cloves, crushed

2 tablespoons hazelnut butter

2 tablespoons freshly squeezed lemon juice

2 tablespoons chopped parsley

1 Cut aubergines in half lengthways. Put them in the oven at 425 degrees for 35–45 minutes, depending on size and thickness of aubergine. You'll want to line your baking pan with foil as aubergines do release liquid that can burn on the pan. Once baked, you can just turn off the oven and let the whole thing cool for 20–30 minutes. Then the insides willingly come out and are all nice and soft.

2 Scoop the soft pulp out of the skin. Place the pulp in a sieve and, using the back of a spoon, press out the juices.

3 Transfer the aubergine pulp to a blender, add all the remaining ingredients and purée until smooth.

4 Serve with organic pitta bread and vegetable crudités.

Per serving: Calories 75 (From Fat 32); Fat 4 g (Saturated 0 g); Cholesterol 0 mg; Sodium 5 mg; Carbohydrate 11 g (Dietary Fibre 4 g); Protein 2 g.

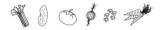

Smoked Mackerel Pâté

This is prime heart and brain food, due to its rich supply of essential fatty acids. It tastes wonderful, too! Serve with a few leaves of any sort of salad that take your fancy, as they all supply you with extra nutrients and chlorophyll.

Preparation time: *1 hour*

Serves: *2–3 as a starter, more if served as a party dip*

250 grams (10 ounces) ready-to-use smoked organic mackerel

150 millilitres (5 fluid ounces) reduced-fat fromage frais

1 tablespoon chopped fresh parsley

1 dessertspoon chopped fresh coriander

Freshly ground pepper and sea salt to taste

Juice of half a lemon

Fresh lemon quarters for serving

1 Using a fork or your fingers, flake the mackerel into small pieces in a bowl.

2 Combine the remaining ingredients and then add the fish gently so it doesn't fall apart and mash into the cheese. Refrigerate for an hour so that the mixture firms up.

3 Serve with toasted organic sour dough bread and of course – with its Scottish overtones – it's excellent with organic oatcakes.

Per serving: Calories 370 (From Fat 151); Fat 17 g (Saturated 9 g); Cholesterol 106 mg; Sodium 2,885 mg; Carbohydrate 4 g (Dietary Fibre 0g); Protein 44 g. Based on 2 servings.

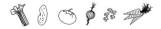

Tapenade

Tapenade is a rich olive spread that is very popular in the Mediterranean where people suffer less heart and cardiovascular disease than in Britain. The olives and oils provide mono-unsaturated fatty acids, and the anchovies supply Omega 3 oils, to combat furred arteries and enhance your detox-busting immune system.

Speciality tools: *Food processor or blender*

Preparation time: *15 minutes*

Serves: *2–3*

20 to 30 pitted large green or black olives (or a mixture of both), coarsely chopped

1 tablespoon capers, rinsed, drained, and chopped

1 t fresh lime juice

3 teaspoons organic olive oil

4 to 5 anchovies, drained and chopped

2–3 grinds of cracked black pepper

1 Put all ingredients in a blender or food processor and whisk for a minute or two, until everything is blended.

2 It's nicest chilled, so refrigerate for an hour or two, or until you're ready to tuck in. Then use as spread or dip, and enjoy.

Per serving: *Calories 178 (From Fat 158); Fat 18 g (Saturated 1 g); Cholesterol 7 mg; Sodium 1,552 mg; Carbohydrate 5 g (Dietary Fibre 0 g); Protein 3 g.*

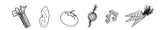

Chapter 17

Vegetarian Detox Dinners

In This Chapter

▶ Finding good value in vegetables

▶ Knowing how to bring out the best in your broccoli (and other veg)

▶ Making tasty and healthy dinners

*W*henever you have your main meal of the day, but particularly if you have it in the evening, during detox you probably look forward to it even more than usual, especially if you are accustomed to snacking during the day.

I urge you to try all of the recipes that follow, even if you don't eat vegetarian fare as a matter of course, because they are kind to the taste buds, provide excellent nutritional value, and have real detox cleansing properties.

Valuing Vegetables

First to choose on a vegetarian regimen (as part of a detox session) are all the commonplace vegetables most of us eat daily or weekly and some of the rarer varieties that carnivores eat only on occasion. Good examples include tomatoes, aubergines, courgettes, sweet potatoes, cabbage, and broccoli.

Bright green veg tend to contain a good supply of vitamins C and bioflavonoids (both powerful antioxidants), which strengthen the immune system during a detox. The rest all contain health-giving plant factors such as the lycopene (cancer-fighting agent) in tomatoes, while cabbage offers the stomach-ulcer-healing vitamin 'U', broccoli is considered a super-food because of its rich supply of antioxidants, and sweet potatoes add bulk and appetite-satisfying properties to a meal without raising your blood sugar too quickly or steeply.

Nearly all fresh plant food is rich in vitamins, minerals and trace elements, and, of course, antioxidants. The potent nutritional elements combat the effect of free radicals (the over-active oxygen molecules sometimes produced by the tissues in excessively high numbers that attack the immune system and other organs and cause a great deal of harm to the immune defence system), individual organs and systems, and the skin on the face where they cause premature ageing signs including deeply entrenched lines and wrinkles.

Foods to avoid are non-organic, old or stale plant foods and any produce containing colouring matter, preservatives, or any other kind of additive.

Preparing Veg

First, try to obtain all the veg you eat in its organic and healthiest state. Frozen and tinned vegetables have a part to play in a detox eating regimen providing they are free from added salt, sugar, and artificial chemicals; but fresh from the ground in which the plants grew, has to be best.

When you boil veg, follow Delia Smith's advice and use the minimum water required for cooking, while ensuring that the vegetables are left on the heat only long enough to soften them acceptably. This means that minimum nutrients are lost during the cooking process, or destroyed by the application of high temperatures.

Similarly, when stir-frying use the least amount of oil consistent with proper cooking, and heat only to the temperature – and for long enough – to ensure that your vegetables are properly cooked.

Treat tinned or frozen fats in the same way. Heat for the minimum time, using the smallest possible quantity of plant oil, although you have to heat stir-fry meals to a moderately high temperature for them to cook at all. Just bear in mind the tender nutrients within the food you are cooking, and handle them with the consideration they deserve!

Cooking Vegetarian Dishes

Please do not be afraid of the word 'vegetarian'! Far from implying a bizarre diet and even more bizarre advocates, vegetarian foods and cooking are set to figure ever more notably in our everyday diet. With the worries presently entertained about the safety of beef and even lamb, and the possible toxin content of sea and river fish, we would all do well to turn earlier rather than later to the vegetarian eating system which, incidentally, wins over thousands of enthusiasts every year from the ranks of die-hard carnivores (meat eaters).

Essentially, if you already like vegetables, then you will find the following vegetarian recipes inspirational. If you don't like vegetables, you're in an even more enviable position! *Now* is the time to set a prejudice or two aside and experiment with an open mind the vegetarian recipes in this chapter.

Onion Pitta Pizza

You may be surprised to find a pizza recipe among detox dinners, but providing you choose good ingredients, you can get away with creating a delicious and wholesome meal that aids detox and is filling and satisfying as well. The tomatoes in the recipe provide lycopene and the olive oil provides mono-unsaturated fatty acids, beneficial to the heart and cardiovascular system.

Preparation time: *20 minutes*

Cooking time: *20–30 minutes*

Serves: *2–4*

4 tablespoons extra virgin organic olive oil

750 grams (1½ pounds) organic onions thinly sliced

4 organic pitta breads

½ cup of organic tomato salsa, divided into four portions

8 black or green olives, pitted and cut in two, divided into four portions

8 sun-dried tomatoes cut in two, divided into four portions

2 tablespoons of chopped fresh basil or oregano, divided into four portions

125 grams (5 ounces) organic mozzarella cheese, shredded, divided into four portions

(continued)

(continued)

1 Heat the oil in a frying pan and sauté the onions over a medium heat for 10–20 minutes, until tender and golden.

2 Place the pitta bread on a baking sheet, spread one portion of tomato salsa evenly to cover each piece. Divide the onions on the pitta breads and on top of them arrange portions of the olives, tomatoes, and fresh herbs. Place a portion of mozzarella slices on top.

3 Bake at 200°C for 10 minutes. Remove from the oven, cut into wedges, and serve.

Per serving: Calories 500 (From Fat 219); Fat 24 g (Saturated 7 g); Cholesterol 28 mg; Sodium 853 mg; Carbohydrate 56 g (Dietary Fibre 5 g); Protein 16 g. Based on 4 servings.

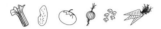

Stir-fry Brussels Sprouts in Plum Sauce

Brussels sprouts are notorious for being hated but, like most victims, many people have more than a kind word to say on their behalf. If you like them, you should enjoy this recipe, which makes use of fresh Brussels sprouts in their prime and brings out their flavour with the help of plum sauce.

Preparation time: *10 minutes*

Cooking time: *10 minutes*

Serves: *2–3*

500 grams (1pound) Brussels sprouts

2 tablespoons olive oil

2 cloves garlic

1 red or yellow pepper

100 grams (4 ounces) mangetout

100 grams (4 ounces) mushrooms – any type you choose from the wide selection available.

6–7 spring onions, trimmed and chopped

1 tablespoon chopped fresh coriander

1 tablespoon plum sauce

1 Trim Brussels sprouts and cut them in half. Cut the pepper into strips. Top and tail the mangetout. Rinse the mushrooms, pat them dry and cut them in half. Crush the garlic.

2 Heat the oil in a wok or large frying pan. Sauté the Brussels sprouts, mushrooms and pepper for 2 minutes.

3 Add the mangetout, mushrooms, garlic, spring onions and coriander.

4 Continue cooking for 2–3 minutes, then place everything in a bowl and add the plum sauce and stir.

Per serving: Calories 148 (From Fat 69); Fat 8 g (Saturated 1 g); Cholesterol 0 mg; Sodium 56 mg; Carbohydrate 19 g (Dietary Fibre 5 g); Protein 5 g. Based on 4 servings.

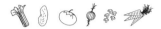

Swede Patties

You may look at the Brussels sprout recipe preceding this, and then at this one and decide that vegetarian food is not for you. I urge you to try both, the present recipe being deliciously flavoured with sesame seeds and supplying beta-carotene, natural fibre, and both vitamin C and bioflavonoids.

Preparation time: *10–15 minutes*

Cooking time: *20 minutes*

Serves: *4*

750 grams (1½ lbs) swede, peeled and chopped into 2–3 centimetre pieces.

250 grams (½ lb) potatoes, chopped into 2–3 centimetre pieces.

1 organic egg

2 cups organic wholemeal flour, divided

1 tablespoon chopped fresh parsley

2 tablespoons organic sesame seeds

Pepper to taste

2 tablespoons organic, cold-pressed, vegetable margarine

1 tablespoon organic sunflower oil

1 tablespoon sesame oil

1 Boil the swede and potatoes together for 20 minutes, until very tender. Drain, then mash them with a hand masher. Add the egg and 1 cup of wholemeal flour and the herbs and blend for 2–3 minutes. Pour out into a bowl and stir in the sesame seeds and pepper.

2 Place the remaining cup of flour in a shallow container and spoon ¼ cup of the swede and potato mixture onto the flour. Using well-floured hands, shape the mixture into a rissole (small cake), coating it thoroughly with the flour. Repeat with the remaining mixture.

(continued)

(continued)

3 Heat the margarine and oils in a large frying pan over a medium heat. Gently lift the swede and potato patties and cook for 3 minutes on each side, turning once.

4 Drain on absorbent paper and serve in wholemeal roll with a green leaf salad.

Per serving: *Calories 473 (From Fat 156); Fat 17 g (Saturated 3 g); Cholesterol 53 mg; Sodium 491 mg; Carbohydrate 70 g (Dietary Fibre 12 g); Protein 14 g.*

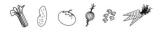

Vegetable Pasta

Do try this vegetable pasta, which is filling, nutritious and very palatable because the fresh vegetables complement the wholewheat pasta and vice versa. You are being supplied with a low-G.I., high-fibre meal, a selection of delicious fresh vegetables and some low-fat dairy, flavoured with parmesan cheese and chopped chives.

Preparation time: *20 minutes*

Cooking time: *25 minutes*

Serves: *4–6*

2 tablespoons organic olive oil	*Salt and freshly ground black pepper to taste*
2 onions, thinly sliced	
2 cloves of garlic, crushed	*100 grams (4 ounces) of low-fat fromage frais*
1 cup of small cauliflower florets	*500 grams (1 pound) wholewheat pasta of choice, cooked*
2 courgettes, sliced	
2 stalks of celery, sliced	*Grated organic parmesan cheese to cover*
4 tomatoes, peeled and chopped	
½ teaspoon of mixed herbs	*Chopped chives as garnish*

1 Heat the oil in a large frying pan or wok. Sauté the onions and garlic until the onion is tender. Add the cauliflower, courgettes and celery and sauté for 2 minutes. Blend in the tomatoes, herbs and seasoning, and cook for a further 2 minutes.

3 Cook until tender, and stir in the fromage frais. Heat thoroughly.

4 Add the hot pasta to the sauce, combine thoroughly and sprinkle with Parmesan and chives. Serve with crusty sourdough bread.

Per serving: Calories 450 (From Fat 100); Fat 11 g (Saturated 5 g); Cholesterol 24 mg; Sodium 223 mg; Carbohydrate 76 g (Dietary Fibre 14 g); Protein 18 g. Based on 6 servings.

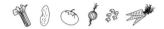

Mumbles Leek Tart

This tart is quite delicious and popular in many parts of Wales, including the Gower Peninsula. It pays to buy leeks at their freshest, when the vegetables are firm to the touch and the green area is bright and juicy. This recipe supplies the following nutrients: chlorophyll (a powerful anti-oxidant), Omega-6 fatty acids, vitamin E and plenty of fibre.

Specialty tools: *25 centimetres (9 inch) flan tin*

Preparation time: *30 minutes*

Cooking time: *40–50 minutes*

Serves: *6–8*

1000 grams (2½ pounds) leeks

60 grams (2 ounces) organic, cold-pressed margarine

1–2 tablespoons flour

Salt and black pepper

2 organic eggs, beaten

1 tablespoon organic low-fat crème fraîche or the top of organic milk, plus two tablespoons to finish

200–340 grams (8–12 ounces) organic shortcrust wholemeal pastry. (You can make this yourself or buy it from a health food shop.)

Lemon juice

1 Wash and chop the leeks, slicing carefully down between the envelope layers and discarding the upper part where the green section runs into the coarse fibrous end.

2 Heat the margarine in a frying pan or wok, then add the leeks and cook until they soften. When the leeks are soft and tender (5–10 mins), add a generous lump of the margarine and leave to stew a few minutes longer.

(continued)

(continued)

3 Take the leeks off the heat and add just enough flour. Mix them well together, then season with the salt and black pepper. Stir in the beaten eggs and the crème fraîche or top of the milk, forming a thick mush.

4 Line the flan tin with the pastry and spread the leek mixture over it. Spill over a little more crème fraîche (about 2 tablespoons) and bake in the oven, set at 220°C for 20 minutes. Then lower the heat by a couple of notches (to about 180°C and continue cooking until the pastry is crisp and the top nicely browned. This should take about 20 minutes.

5 Serve with a fresh spinach leaf salad, or fresh watercress. Add a squeeze of lemon juice to the tart just before serving.

Per serving: Calories 380 (From Fat 240); Fat 27 g (Saturated 9 g); Cholesterol 73 mg; Sodium 292 mg; Carbohydrate 28 g (Dietary Fibre 5 g); Protein 7 g. Based on 6 servings.

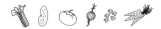

Spaghetti with Tomato Salsa and Oregano

This is a very filling recipe and well worth preparing for yourself alone or for two or three guests. The tomato supplies lycopene and the garlic and oregano make a flavourful recipe.

Preparation time: *10–15 mins.*

Cooking time: *15–20 mins.*

Serves: *2*

3 tablespoons extra virgin olive oil

2 onion, peeled and thinly sliced

2 garlic clove, chopped

12 tablespoons organic tomato salsa

200 millilitres (7 fluid ounces) organic tomato juice

20 black or green olives, stoned and chopped

2 tablespoon of fresh oregano

Freshly ground black pepper

450 grams (1pound) wholemeal spaghetti

Sprigs of oregano to garnish

1 Heat the oil in a frying pan and sauté the onion and the garlic until beginning to colour. This should take about 5 minutes. Add the tomato salsa and tomato juice and simmer gently for 8–10 minutes, stirring occasionally. Add the olives and oregano and simmer for a further 10 minutes. Season well with black pepper.

2 Meanwhile, cook the pasta in plenty of boiling water until *al dente* (pasta is still slightly firm and not totally soft). Drain and toss immediately in the sauce, garnishing with oregano leaves before serving.

Per serving: Calories 485 (From Fat 74); Fat 8 g (Saturated 1 g); Cholesterol 0 mg; Sodium 356 mg; Carbohydrate 92 g (Dietary Fibre 15 g); Protein 18 g. Based on 4 servings.

Stir-fried Broccoli, Mushrooms, and Cashew Nuts

This delicious recipe delivers the benefits of lightly cooked broccoli and mushrooms, which supply protein, and cashew nuts that supply Omega-6 essential fatty acids.

Preparation time: *10 minutes*

Cooking time: *10–15 minutes*

Serves: *4*

2 tablespoons organic oil, for example sunflower oil or peanut oil

100 grams (4 ounces) unsalted cashew nuts

1 head of broccoli, divided into florets

2–3 heads of baby bok choy, washed and thickly sliced

210-gram (9-ounce) can of organic straw mushrooms, drained

1 onion sliced

2 tablespoons organic soy sauce

1 Heat the oil in a frying pan and fry the cashews until golden. This will take about 3 minutes. Remove from heat and set aside.

2 In the same pan as you used for the nuts, add the bok choy, onion and broccoli and stir-fry it until tender but still crisp.

3 Add the mushrooms, the cashews, and the soy sauce. Stir and toss until heated through.

Per serving: Calories 261 (From Fat 174); Fat 19 g (Saturated 3 g); Cholesterol 0 mg; Sodium 703 mg; Carbohydrate 16 g (Dietary Fibre 5 g); Protein 10 g.

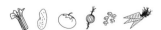

Chickpea Curry

Chickpea curry may not sound terribly exciting if you are not familiar with chickpeas, but they have an excellent nutty flavour and a crunchy texture maintained throughout the cooking process. This recipe, therefore, gives you lots of fibre, lycopene from the tomato paste and the cancer-fighting benefits of turmeric.

Preparation time: *20 minutes*

Cooking time: *30 minutes*

Serves: *6*

2 tablespoons organic safflower or sunflower oil

2 onions, finely chopped

2 garlic cloves, chopped

1 tablespoon ground coriander

1 teaspoon mild chilli powder

2 teaspoons turmeric

3 tablespoons sun-dried tomato paste

300 grams (11 ounces) potatoes, peeled and cut into bite-sized chunks

400-gram (14-ounce) can of chopped tomatoes

1 litre (1¾ pints) hot vegetable stock

250 grams (9 ounces) of green beans or peas

2 x 400-gram (14-ounce) cans of chickpeas, drained

1 Heat the oil in a pan, fry the onion until golden, then add the garlic, spices, and tomato paste. Cook gently for 2–3 minutes, stirring.

2 Add the potatoes, the tomatoes, and the stock and season with a very little sea salt and freshly ground pepper. Cover and bring to the boil, then simmer, half covered, for 20 minutes.

3 Add the green beans or peas, and the chickpeas. Cook for a further 5–10 minutes.

Per serving: *Calories 281 (From Fat 66); Fat 7 g (Saturated 1 g); Cholesterol 0 mg; Sodium 1,239 mg; Carbohydrate 45 g (Dietary Fibre 10 g); Protein 12 g.*

Chapter 18

Fish and Fowl Detox Dinners

In This Chapter

▶ Choosing Fish and Fowl

▶ Fishing for a healthy detox

▶ Tucking in with the birds

*P*rotein is a vital nutrient supporting health and life; it is especially necessary during the middle and late stages of a detox programme, when the body is regaining energy and starting to renew worn out cells.

Choosing Fish and Fowl

Healthy protein can be obtained from combining the grains, cereals, pulses and nuts of vegetarian meals. However, detox is not about turning your back on animal protein unless you choose to do so. Good sources of animal protein include both fish and fowl, as you will see in the following section.

Talking about fish

Fish contains up to 60 per cent first class protein. It contains hardly any saturated fat, and so-called flat fish such as plaice and skate, and others like cod and haddock are very low in fat generally.

Oily fish, however, are rich in omega-3 fatty acids (Read more about this in Chapter 5), and therefore contribute to your health and detox in two ways – they provide first-class protein, and also boost your heart, circulatory system and brain.

Popular oily fish include salmon, mackerel, sardines, halibut, herrings, and whitebait.

Seafood – prawns in particular – are often shunned by health fanatics because of their cholesterol content. However, the actual quantity of cholesterol you would be likely to obtain from 4–6 ounces (100–150 g) of prawns, or shrimps, mussels, whelks, scallops and the like, is relatively small.

My advice is enjoy it during your detox when you feel in need of a treat – just make sure you check its origins and that the creature comes from safe (uncontaminated) fresh or seawater. It must not, of course, ever have seen artificial colouring or chemical additives of any other kind.

Fish has generally delicate flesh that responds well to gentle steaming, baking or medium-temperature microwaving. Don't boil a fish like plaice or whiting for example, as it will disintegrate into small fragments. And while you can use a little cold-pressed olive or other cooking plant oil for stir-frying fish, do not on any account – while detoxing – dip it in batter and deep-fry it! Don't cook it in butter or other no-no oils and fats either.

Going for the birds

There is less to say about the nutritional benefits of poultry and fowl (game birds), simply because they are not sources of healthy polyunsaturated fats. That said, however, they contain far less fat than most red meat, and that which is present can be more easily avoided (because it is mainly found just under the skin). Farmed red meat is 'marbled', which means it has thin streaks of saturated fat running all the way through it, interspersed with its red, non-fatty flesh.

Make sure you remember how much fat there can be in chicken, turkey and other birds. We no longer dive our fingers inside to rescue giblets for gravy, so it's easy to disregard all the bits you cannot see. While a whole bird is being roasted, the interior fat of course melts, and mixes with the delicious meat juices, eventually setting with them into a jelly.

If you roast a bird, make certain that you avoid as much fat as possible. And avoid eating ducks, geese, and other waterfowl as they are overloaded with subcutaneous (below-skin) fat to protect their body heat from chilling in cold water.

Chicken, turkey, and other dry-ish edible birds such as wood pigeon, snipe, and grouse are delicious, possibly unfamiliar, and loaded with first-class protein. They also supply the mood-balancing amino acid, tryptophan, making them an excellent choice if you are depressed or down.

When roasting poultry and fowl use the minimum (or preferably no) additional fat or oil; or buy chicken breasts, for example, that contain plenty of vital amino acids and virtually no fat. Detox-friendly cooking methods for low-fat bird meat include stir-frying in small strips, baking in a covered dish or foil parcel in a moderate oven, and dry-frying – using a dry, heated frying pan, or work to sear the meat and seal in the juices, then cook it slowly until cooked all the way through.

Cooking with Fish and Fowl

Here you will find a good selection of fish and fowl main dishes, with some of which you may have been long familiar, and with others perhaps offering a surprise flavour combination. Chicken and lemon go well together, for example, and chopped chicken with left-over veg can form the basis of a cooked light meal or supper. Bon appetite!

Chicken Omelette

This is an ideal omelette to make on Monday, when you may not feel like cooking, but have a leftover chicken facing you, following the Sunday roast. The chicken is a good source of tryptophan amino acid, which boosts mood and allays anxiety. The olive oil is an excellent source of mono-unsaturated fatty acids, which enhance heart health, and the organic eggs supply first-class protein and a range of vitamins and minerals.

Preparation time: *10 minutes*

Cooking time: *4–5 minutes*

Serves: *1*

1–2 teaspoon of organic olive oil

2 organic eggs

Salt and pepper to taste

85 grams (3 ounces) sliced, cooked chicken

1 teaspooon of cold, cooked garden peas or other veg in bite-size pieces

1 tablespoon of finely chopped cooked potato

(continued)

(continued)

1 Heat the olive oil in a frying pan. Meanwhile, beat the eggs in a bowl and season with a little salt and freshly ground black pepper.

2 Once the oil is hot, pour the beaten eggs into the pan, tilting it so that the eggs cover the base. Cook for 2–3 minutes until the omelette is cooked underneath.

3 Place the chicken and vegetables in the centre of the omelette, fold over and continue cooking until the whole omelette is heated through.

Per serving: Calories 319 (From Fat 138); Fat 15 g (Saturated 4 g); Cholesterol 497 mg; Sodium 193 mg; Carbohydrate 3 g (Dietary Fibre 0 g); Protein 39 g.

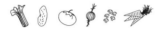

Spicy Lime Swordfish

This is as delicious as it sounds. The fish is an excellent source of protein and omega-3 fatty acids. The lime zest provides vitamin C and bioflavonoids and the garlic enhances your digestive processes.

Preparation time: *10 minutes*

Marinade time: *2 hours*

Cooking time: *6–7 minutes*

Serves: *4*

2½ centimetres (1 inch) fresh ginger root

2 tablespoons of extra virgin olive oil

Juice and zest of one lime and 1 lime sliced into rounds

2 garlic cloves, crushed

4 x 150-gram (6-ounce) swordfish steaks

Freshly ground pepper to taste

1 Peel and finely grate the ginger root. Press it in a large shallow dish together with the oil, the juice and zest of the lime, and the garlic. Stir it round and lay the swordfish steaks in it. Marinade for 45 minutes on each side.

2 Pre-heat a griddle pan. Lift the swordfish steaks out of the marinade and place them in the pan. Season with a little freshly ground pepper. Cook the steaks over a low heat for 2–3 minutes on each side. After turning them for the final time, place a slice or two of lime on top and cook for a further 1–2 minutes until the fish is opaque.

Per serving: Calories 255 (From Fat 118); Fat 13 g (Saturated 3 g); Cholesterol 62 mg; Sodium 143 mg; Carbohydrate 1 g (Dietary Fibre 0 g); Protein 32 g.

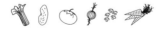

Devilled Chicken Burgers

This chicken recipe also provides tryptophan amino acids and lycopene-rich tomato paste. The Worcestershire sauce peps up the taste, giving it a pleasant and healthy zest.

Preparation time: *15 minutes*

Cooking time: *15 minutes*

Serves: *4*

450 grams (1 pound) lean, freshly-minced raw chicken

2 very finely chopped shallots

½ teaspoon (or a large pinch) mixed herbs

1 dessertspoon of sun-dried tomato paste

1 organic egg, beaten

1 tablespoon of organic Worcestershire sauce

1 Place the chicken in a bowl, together with the shallots, herbs, tomato paste, beaten egg, and Worcestershire sauce. Mix together.

2 Wet your hands to shape the mixture into four round patties, about 2½ centimetres (1 inch) thick.

3 Preheat the grill and cook the burgers for 5–7 minutes on each side.

4 Serve with fresh green beans.

Per serving: *Calories 127 (From Fat 57); Fat 6 g (Saturated 2 g); Cholesterol 95 mg; Sodium 95 mg; Carbohydrate 6 g (Dietary Fibre 0 g); Protein 13 g. Analysed without beans.*

Prawns with Soy Sauce

If you love prawns, eating them during detox can provide a pleasant treat. Prawns are a good source of protein, and the brightly coloured vegetables in this recipe supply lots of vitamin C and a range of other vitamins and minerals.

Preparation time: *5 minutes*

Cooking time: *5–7 minutes*

Serves: *4*

2 tablespoons soy sauce

6 tablespoons cider vinegar

2 teaspoon of organic maple syrup

6 spring onions, trimmed and finely chopped

2 teaspoons vegetable oil

300 grams (11½ ounces) raw peeled tiger prawns

6 small carrots, washed, trimmed, and thinly sliced

3–4 heads of baby bok choy, trimmed and thinly sliced

1 Place the soy sauce in a dish together with the cider vinegar, maple syrup, and spring onions. Combine and set aside.

2 Steam the prawns for 3–4 minutes until pink and opaque, then toss in the set aside dressing.

3 Heat the oil in a frying pan or wok. Add the carrots and bok choy, stir-frying until tender. Allow about 4 minutes for tender, crisp vegetables. Add the prawns, together with the sauce, stir well and serve.

Per serving: *Calories 147 (From Fat 30); Fat 3 g (Saturated 0 g); Cholesterol 121 mg; Sodium 658 mg; Carbohydrate 14 g (Dietary Fibre 4 g); Protein 16 g.*

Lime and Coriander Turkey Breasts

Turkeys are as freely available as chickens nowadays and are an even richer source of the amino acid tryptophan. Fresh lime complements the flavour of the meat and, together with the herbs, provides a range of bioflavonoids, chlorophyll, vitamin C, and other nutrients.

Preparation time: *20 minutes*

Cooking time: *20–30 minutes*

Serves: *4*

125 millilitres (4 fluid ounces) fresh lime juice

Zest of 1 lime

2 tablespoons of chopped fresh parsley

2 tablespoons of chopped fresh coriander leaves

1 tablespoon of extra virgin olive oil

1 garlic clove, pressed

Salt and pepper to taste

120–180 grams (4–6 ounces) skinless turkey-breast fillet per person

1 Pre-heat the oven to 200°C.

2 Place the lime juice and zest in a bowl and whisk it together with the chopped herbs, the oil, and the garlic clove. Season with salt and pepper to taste.

3 Slash the turkey breasts several times to open them up slightly, and place in an ovenproof dish.

4 Pour over the marinade and top each turkey breast with a small wedge of lime or extra zest.

5 Cook for 30–40 minutes, or until cooked through.

Per serving: *Calories 161 (From Fat 37); Fat 4 g (Saturated 1 g); Cholesterol 74 mg; Sodium 48 mg; Carbohydrate 3 g (Dietary Fibre 0 g); Protein 27 g.*

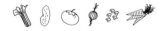

Spaghetti with Mussel Sauce

Providing you are not allergic to wheat, there is no reason why you shouldn't have at least one pasta dish while detoxing. Choose the organic sort made from wholewheat, which is a rich source of fibre and nutrients, and pick very fresh mussels, that have not been immersed in vinegar. The mussels provide both a delicious taste and a source of protein and the whole dish is filling and satisfying.

Preparation time: *15 minutes*

Cooking time: *About 30 minutes*

Serves: *4*

2 teaspoons of olive oil

1 onion, finely chopped

3 garlic cloves, finely chopped

400 grams (14 ounces) cherry tomatoes, halved

2 x 200-gram (7-ounce) cans of mussels in brine, drained and rinsed to remove the salt

2 tablespoons of freshly chopped parsley

228 grams (8 ounces) of wholewheat spaghetti

1 Heat the oil in a frying pan, add the onion and fry gently for 5–10 minutes until soft. Add the garlic and cook gently for a further 2 minutes.

2 Add the cherry tomatoes to the pan and stir in the mussels together with the parsley. Season to taste and remove from the heat. Keep warm.

3 Meanwhile cook the spaghetti in a large pan of boiling salted water, according to packet instructions. Drain, then toss through the sauce. Serve with wilted (lightly cooked – about 2 minutes in boiling water) spinach or a green salad.

Per serving: *Calories 421 (From Fat 71); Fat 8 g (Saturated 1 g); Cholesterol 56 mg; Sodium 384 mg; Carbohydrate 57 g (Dietary Fibre 9 g); Protein 33 g. Analysed with fresh mussels.*

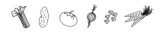

Almond and Apricot Chicken

Almond and apricot are a classic combination and go very well with chicken, other poultry, and many fish dishes. The apricots supply vitamin C and beta-carotene, and the almonds supply essential oils and boost the fibre content contributed by the wholegrain rice.

Preparation/Cooking time: *30–40 minutes*

Serves: *2*

30 grams (1ounce) flaked almonds

120 grams (4 ounces) easy-cook wholegrain rice

Salt and pepper

2 teaspoons vegetable oil

1 medium onion, finely chopped

200 grams (7 ounce) skinless chicken breasts, cut into 2½ centimetre (1 inch) pieces

½ teaspoon of ground cinnamon

30 grams (1 ounce) ready-to-eat organic dried apricots, each cut into four

1 tablespoon of chopped, fresh parsley

1 Heat a thick-based frying pan and dry-fry the almonds until they change colour (don't burn!). Remove the almonds from the pan and set aside.

2 Put the rice into a large pan of boiling, lightly salted water, and cook until tender (25–30 minutes). Meanwhile, heat the oil in the frying pan, add the onion and cook gently for 5–6 minutes until softened.

3 Turn the heat up slightly, and add the chicken, stir-frying briskly to seal the pieces all over. Reduce the heat, and cook gently keeping covered for 10 minutes, stirring occasionally.

4 Add the cinnamon and apricots, stir and cook gently for 5 minutes.

5 When the rice is cooked, drain and rinse with freshly-boiled water and drain again thoroughly. Tip the hot rice into the pan with the other ingredients, stir well, season to taste and cook for 2–3 minutes, stirring constantly.

6 Just before serving, stir in the toasted almonds, reserving a few to scatter on top. Decorate with the freshly chopped parsley and serve at once.

Per serving: Calories 493 (From Fat 143); Fat 16 g (Saturated 2 g); Cholesterol 65 mg; Sodium 349 mg; Carbohydrate 56 g (Dietary Fibre 6 g); Protein 31 g.

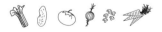

Smoked Haddock with Broad Beans, Spinach and Sweet Corn

Sometimes, especially when dining alone, you want your detox dinner to be simple, straightforward, and easy to prepare. This recipe fits the bill. Make sure that the haddock is properly smoked and not coloured.

Haddock is not especially rich in essential oils, but it provides filling and tasty protein. The spinach is rich in fibre and minerals to boost your gut and immune defence system. The broad beans provide a range of anti-oxidant nutrients for the same purpose.

Preparation/Cooking time: *15–20 minutes*

Serves: *1*

120–175 grams (4–6 ounces) smoked haddock

120–175g (4–6 ounces) fresh organic spinach

2 heaped tablespoons of organic broad beans, frozen or fresh

100 grams (3½ ounces) baby sweet corn

1 Place the haddock on a microwave-proof plate. Pour over a tablespoon of water, cover, and microwave on medium power for 3–4 minutes, until flesh is opaque. (Smoked haddock is semi-cooked and slightly opaque – some people eat it like this, but cooking is best in this recipe.)

2 Wash spinach, shake off excess water, and wilt over a medium heat in a saucepan.

3 Tip the beans into a small saucepan of boiling lightly-salted water and cook until pleasantly soft or *al dente*, according to taste.

4 Meanwhile, heat the baby sweet corn in a small quantity of boiling, lightly-salted water for 2–3 minutes, until soft or *al dente*.

5 Drain everything that requires draining, place the fish onto a warmed plate, top with spinach, and scatter the beans and sweet corn. Sit back and enjoy your feast.

Per serving: *Calories 258 (From Fat 18); Fat 2 g (Saturated 0 g); Cholesterol 87 mg; Sodium 1,069 mg; Carbohydrate 29 g (Dietary Fibre 8 g); Protein 35 g.*

Part VI
The Part of Tens

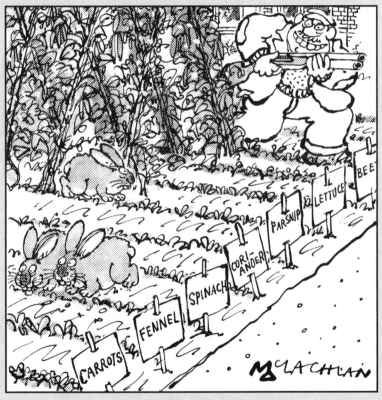

"Spinach, carrots, parsnips, it's what humans call detox, for a long & healthy life."

In this part . . .

*I*n this part you'll find three chapters giving you ten tips for getting the most from the detox process. I describe ten complementary therapies that can help your body cleanse itself and revitalise itself afterwards, ten myths that surround detox, and ten tips to boost your motivation to try the detox process – and keep going once you have taken the plunge! I finish with a list of healthy foods and the benefits they give you.

Chapter 19

Ten Therapies that Enhance Detox

*M*ost people use some form of complementary therapy, even if they don't think of it as such. Camphorated oil was a popular nineteenth century remedy for chesty coughs, and it gave way to preparations such as 'Vic' during the twentieth century. Mothers have been rubbing this and similar remedies on babies' and children's chests for many decades, without thinking of it in terms of aromatherapy. Our grandparents, great-grandparents, and probably several generations of grandparents before them used the medicinal herb senna in some form for the relief of constipation. It is used just as much today, 'Sennokot' tablets forming the mainstay of lazy bowel treatment for many. You're probably also familiar with acupuncture, whose renown has increased prolifically since the 1960s, although it is an ages-old treatment technique, originating with the ancient Chinese several thousand years B.C.

You can use these and other complementary therapies and remedies to effectively enhance the detox process, and likewise to relieve some of the symptoms you may experience as toxins are cleansed from your system and your organs are balanced and reinvigorated by the detox.

The following ten therapies are simply examples of many you may choose to use for yourself. There is a great deal of information to be found in books, leaflets, and on the Internet about the use of simple, readily-available remedies, all of which can be accessed through pharmacists and health food shops.

On the Health Scent with Aromatherapy

Aromatherapy oils are the pure essences of plants and as such have been used (probably) for thousands of years to enhance energy and well-being and to relieve minor disorders. Ancient uses included massages to relieve sore or torn muscles and joints, and poultices and compresses for the treatment of infected and inflamed areas and wounds and other trauma.

One beneficial use of aromatherapy during detox is in the form of steam inhalation. The process is simple and the only ingredient you need to purchase is the aromatherapy oil itself, such as:

- Tea-tree oil or essence of eucalyptus and rosemary improve the cleansing of your lungs and upper airways, helping rid them of excess mucus, dead cells, and other inhaled toxins.

- Essence of peppermint is beneficial for the digestive tract and the airways and lungs and it also has a reviving effect and can help to relieve fatigue, headache, and migraine.

- Rose essence is richly floral and feminine, and is a good remedy for female problems such as menstrual disorders which you might feel more acutely during a detox. It also relieves anxiety and stress, both of which you are attempting to relieve during a detox programme and, in addition, is used by aromatherapists to treat liver congestion.

Follow these steps for an aromatherapy pick-me-up during detox:

1. **Place a medium-sized bowl on a firm surface and fill it with near-boiling water.**

2. **Add four or five drops of chosen oil.**

3. **Place a towel over your head so that it covers your head, neck and the bowl.**

4. **Inhale as slowly and deeply as you find comfortable for five to ten minutes.**

I suggest that you talk to your GP and consider having specialist treatment from a qualified aromatherapist if you are, or suspect you are, suffering from liver damage.

But there is no reason why you should not profit by adding a few drops of pure rose essence either to your bath water or to a steam inhalation.

Continuing the Trend toward Herbs

The medicinal use of herbs is probably the oldest form of treatment known to humans – although our ancestors may well have used massage for sore or injured body parts, while in the process of detecting helpful herbs by trial and error.

Most herbal remedies are available from qualified pharmacists and qualified medical herbalists, both of whom, but especially the latter, are in an ideal position to discuss the uses of such remedies with you.

Make sure you *always* to follow any given directions, including those on the packet label, closely and accurately. The fact that herbal remedies are natural does not in any way render them harmless; the fact that they can and do have profoundly beneficial effects upon many disorders emphasises their potency, which can prove a double-edged sword if they are taken incorrectly.

It is true that many herbal preparations are in theory safer and kinder to the body than occasionally harsh medical drugs and when taken as they should be, are unlikely to cause side-effects.

If you experience adverse symptoms of any sort following a herbal remedy, stop taking it at once and see your medical herbalist or a doctor. Possibilities include a rash, nausea, discomfort of the skin or nasal lining, or headache.

The following are herbal remedies with safe, useful, and healing properties that will aid the detox process and relieve any associated symptoms:

✔ **Senna** relieves constipation and can be taken in the form of a herbal tea or, more commonly, as tablets.

   Senna can cause discomfort and diarrhoea in some sensitive people and you would be better off trying a gentler remedy, such as increasing your fibre intake, if you think you may be susceptible to this.

✔ **Camomile** is a favourite calming herb and the tea soothes the digestion and helps to cure insomnia. Camomile cream or lotion is useful for inflammatory skin conditions – sensitive areas of skin can become inflamed during the detox process while toxins are being shed.

✔ **Aloe vera** provides another useful skin application. The gel can be applied beneficially to inflamed skin conditions and rashes and, in addition, is a useful digestive aid. You are unlikely to experience digestive upsets in response to a detox programme, but you might suffer from mild indigestion, for instance, belching or wind, while your digestive system is in the process of cleansing itself and becoming used to a radical change in diet, and aloe vera can soothe these symptoms

✔ Taking **elderflower** tea at bedtime is a long-established treatment for feverish conditions because elderflower helps the body to sweat. If you use hot spices such as chilli or cayenne pepper during detox to promote sweating, sipping elderflower tea may well enhance these effects. In addition, elderflower herbal preparations can aid the respiratory tract to shed accumulated debris and toxins if taken regularly – a cup twice a day for 2–3 months, for example.

You can buy elderflower tea in sachet form or make it up for yourself, using the dried flowers available from health food shops and herbalists. You can add a slice of lemon or a couple of leaves of mint or lemon balm to elderflower tea, if you find the flavour too bland.

Curing Like with Like in Homeopathy

You may find it difficult to understand precisely how homeopathy works. Its underlying principle that 'like cures like' is a cause of misunderstanding and scepticism, although homeopathy has a long history of success.

Essentially, extremely minute particles of the substance which would normally cause illness or upset when taken in larger quantities, are used to relieve or cure symptoms. Nausea, for example, is relieved by a herbal remedy known as Ipecac, the same substance which in far larger quantities can be used to treat a drug overdose by inducing vomiting.

Two important points about homeopathy are that the remedies have been found to work for many millions of people and are absolutely safe for the treatment of people of all ages, from newborn babies to the very elderly and infirm.

Homeopathic remedies can be found in chemists and health food stores. You take them according to the package instructions which vary with both the remedy and the characteristics and symptoms of the person taking them. However, generally (for tablets) you place one on the tongue and let it melt. Avoid strong-tasting foods and drinks like coffee and peppermint, and also alcohol, before taking them, and handle them as little as possible. The following are likely to prove useful to you during detox:

✔ **Nux vomica** is a good remedy for a hangover or for the symptoms you may experience shortly after giving up alcohol. It also gets rid of nausea and headaches. Nux vomica aids colds, flu and catarrh and, therefore, is useful to the respiratory tract in getting rid of excess mucus. It will prove helpful if you wake up worrying in the middle of the night and also prefer to be left alone when ill.

✔ **Silica** helps the body expel various toxins and foreign bodies, including splinters, dirt from a wound and other debris. It also relieves headaches, especially caused by hunger and accompanied by ringing in the ears.

✔ **Natrum mur** relieves bad headaches that start in the morning where you feel the need to continue to sleep and, possibly, also relieves unexpressed grief. A further symptom may be great thirst with a hot feeling head and a red face, and it aids digestive upsets which include belching and tummy bloating.

✔ **Pulsatilla** can be tried whenever you are feeling low and tearful. Try it too when you are afflicted by heavy mucus in the respiratory tract and a cough that comes on at night. It also relieves moodiness associated with any illness or feeling of weakness – the latter may be a transitory symptom of detox.

Adjusting Your Energies with Ayurveda

The literal meaning of Ayurveda is the science (veda) of long life. The main traditional holistic healing system in use in India, it's based on the belief that well-being is affected by constantly fluctuating vital energies; treatment aims to restore their balance.

Ayurvedic medicine is used to treat a range of illnesses, including arthritis, asthma, heart disease, and many common complaints. Problems particularly relevant to a toxic lifestyle and detoxing include liver disorders, stress, a low mood, fatigue, and skin eruptions.

An Ayurvedic practitioner cleans and detoxifies using massage oils, saunas, and laxatives or enemas.

When feeling toxic or during detox, take 2–4 capsules daily of a standardised extract of gotu kola supplement containing 25 milligrams of triterpenes. The lower dose is appropriate if you are requiring more energy while the higher dose, which can occasionally cause headaches, has a tranquillising effect.

Gotu kola, which contains no caffeine and is not related to the kola nut, helps to relive anxiety and a low mood, assists in maintaining tranquillity once you acquire it, and aids in relaxing muscular tension. It also cleanses the blood and increases stamina and both physical and mental energy.

Drinking Up Juice Therapy

Juicing is tailor-made as a DIY tool for use during detox. For this you need an electric juicer which you can obtain from most electrical and chain stores. You require the kind that will juice any and all fruit and vegetables, giving you access to the full cleansing powers of these foods.

The benefits of fresh fruit and vegetable juices include:

- **Providing fluid:** Fruits and veg are mainly composed of water in their natural state which is a bonus during detox when you need to increase your fluid intake and get tired of drinking plain water. Many juices have a fairly thick consistency and can make you feel quite full and satisfied.

- **Supplying soluble fibres:** Pectin is an example of these useful scavengers of debris and toxins. Fibre then helps to eliminate these toxins from the body. Fruits with a high pectin content include apples, lemons, oranges, and grapefruit, although you may not wish to use grapefruit juice during a detox fast (see Chapter 3 for the reasons).

- **Adding antioxidants:** The 'cavalry' of the nutrient world, antioxidants are probably the most important constituent in fruit and vegetable juices. They gallop through your blood and tissue cells to combat the free radicals that can cause so much tissue harm and damage.

The following list contains just seven of the many juices that you can use, and includes some of their beneficial constituents. Individual plants also have unique phytochemicals with their own cleansing and detoxing properties:

- **Carrot** juice is unequalled for increasing vitality and stamina. It has an antibacterial action and is said to be highly alkaline. It contains 12 minerals including potassium, calcium, phosphorous, and manganese and it is useful when used in conjunction with other juices for aching joints and muscles and a tender liver.

- **Celery** juice has wonderful solvent properties and helps to keep excess calcium in solution. It is therefore thought to work well for high blood pressure and varicose veins, both of which can develop as a result of a toxic lifestyle. It calms the nerves and also has a high content of both iron and magnesium. Some people find it slightly bitter to drink, but mixed with carrot juice it is highly palatable.

✔ **Beetroot** juice contains the vitamins A, B complex, C and E, and minerals and is high in potassium. It also has a high natural sugar content, and tastes delicious on its own or mixed with almost any other juice.

✔ **Radish** juice is very powerful and should never be taken if you have a stomach ulcer or suffer from stomach acid. It tastes quite potent too and is best mixed by adding a small percentage of it to a mixture of other juice drinks. It's a first-class aid to detox because it clears up mucus conditions and also helps to get rid of gallstones – another reflection of a toxic lifestyle.

✔ **Parsley** juice like other green juices is an excellent cleanser, being rich in the antioxidants and detox constituent chlorophyll and is one of the richest vegetable sources of Vitamin A.

✔ **Apple** juice is probably the finest of all the fruit juices for detox and cleansing purposes.

✔ **Pineapple** juice ready-made (commercially) is a pleasant drink. Freshly-juiced pineapple flesh is absolutely delicious. It is useful during detox because it has a diuretic effect increasing the elimination of excess fluid and toxic wastes in the urine and is rich in Vitamin B complex and E. Perhaps it is best known for its enzyme papain, a useful digestive aid. It is particularly useful to relieve any sort of indigestion and also infections and excess mucus of the throat and lung, such as a phlegmy cough and sore throat.

With the exception of radish juice, it's advisable to start with 100 millilitres (4 fluid ounces) 3–4 times a day, singularly or in combination – take in at most 100 millilitres (4 fluid ounces) at a time and gradually increase the quantity once your digestive system has got used to it.

Sticking to Acupuncture

Acupuncture is an ancient therapy originating with the Chinese about 5,000 years ago. It is part of traditional Chinese medicine and like other holistic therapies recognises a fundamental lifeforce, which it terms *chi*. Chi runs freely through the body when you are in a state of healthy harmony and becomes obstructed when toxins accumulate and also when your biological, mental, and emotional faculties are out of balance.

Acupuncture treatment consists of identifying sites of blockage and releasing the obstruction through stimulation at the key points with specially-designed needles.

Any acupuncture treatment given to aid a specific ailment or symptom will, at the same time, exert a detoxifying effect.

Acupuncture using five points on the outer ear (auricular therapy) is often used during and after detox to help overcome cravings, particularly for alcohol, drugs, nicotine, sugar, caffeine, and other unhealthy foods.

Holding Fast to Acupressure

Acupressure, like acupuncture (see the preceding section), takes into account the free motion of chi energy or stagnation of energy held up at various points where toxins and other debris accumulate.

Acupressure helps the detox process by cleansing (shifting toxins) and also balancing energies. You experience the benefits through acupressure's ability to combat inflammation and sore muscles and joints, relieve fatigue and low energy, increase well-being and sense of vitality, and boost the immune defence system – all of which play important roles in the complete detox process.

The following list addresses just a few of the many symptoms of toxicity you can expect to have relieved or removed by acupressure:

- Excess mucus in the nose, ears, throat or stools and sinus congestion
- Bad breath
- Acne, spots, boils, and pimples
- Cough, wheeziness, and sore throat
- Stiff or tight neck and pains running up the neck into the back of the head
- Dry itchy skin and a worsening of skin conditions from which you may already suffer, such as psoriasis and eczema
- Recurrently itchy or red eyes, puffy eyes, dark circles, and bags below the eyes
- Food allergies, nausea, flatulence, digestive upsets, and diarrhoea or constipation
- Swollen ankles due to fluid retention (if you are otherwise well but habitually suffer from swollen ankles or feet, do check with your doctor that no more serious cause may be present)

✔ Other symptoms include flushing, palpitations, rapid pulse, faintness, pins and needles, disturbed or poor quality sleep, and cramp.

You can receive acupressure at the hands of a qualified practitioner, or apply its techniques yourself. Consult an illustrated book about acupressure for a full account of detox-related points.

Eating Nutritionally Balanced Foods

All foods included in this detox regimen cleanse, balance, and reinvigorate, but I am going to mention here some of the major ones and advise you to introduce as many as you can into your diet, obviously when detoxing, but also afterwards, to combat toxic aspects of your lifestyle. Chapters 5 and 6 look respectively at the sort of foods to eat and why and the sort of foods to avoid and why; the list here simply points you in the direction of foods you may not have thought of including in your detox programme for one reason or another.

✔ **Cherries** have a mildly laxative effect, so help the cleansing process of detox and they are also a good source of Vitamin C and potassium. Their phytochemical constituent, ellagic acid, has a unique anti-cancer effect by blocking an enzyme that cancer cells require to multiply. Ellagic acid is also found in raspberries.

✔ **Grapes,** like cherries, also contain ellagic acid. The red variety contain some lycopene, the anti-cancer phytochemical which is prevalent in tomatoes, but both kinds are rich in antioxidants which are said to be more powerful than Vitamins E and C. They are also an excellent source of potassium and trace elements and can help to prevent bloating.

✔ **Rhubarb** is a brilliant laxative and quite delectable if stewed very gently in a little water until soft and allowed to cool in its juices overnight. Like soya, rhubarb is rich in plant oestrogens which may help menopausal and pre-menstrual symptoms.

✔ **Soya** is worth trying for its balancing effect during detox even if you don't fancy the rather bland protein substitutes. Other soya foods such as MISO and soy sauce are rich in taste and quite delectable. Their phytoestrogens offer a great protection against coronary artery disease and a variety of disorders including cancers of male and female reproductive organs.

- ✔ **Green tea** is currently (and deservedly) very popular with detoxers because it's rich in antioxidants and plant chemicals with an anti-cancer effect. Studies suggest that drinking 4–5 cups of tea (preferably green) every day halves the risks of a heart attack.

- ✔ **Sweet potatoes** are extremely pleasant to eat and their bright orange colour confirms their rich source of Vitamin A (beta carotene). They also provide potassium, magnesium, and Vitamin C and their high fibre content makes them a far healthier alternative to white potatoes for general use.

- ✔ **Parsley** is a great cleanser being very rich in chlorophyll and also supplies Vitamin C, iron, and folic acid. It helps to relieve a poor digestion, colic and wind and has a mildly diuretic effect, increasing the output of urine.

Blossoming under Bach Flower Remedies

This complementary treatment was devised by Dr Edward Bach (pronounced *batch*) a medical doctor, bacteriologist, and homeopath who believed that illness was caused by psychological and emotional conflict and that remedies should be directed inwards towards these, rather than outwards at visible physical symptoms. He produced a range of remedies from plant material infused in spring water.

Bach's flower remedies are an ideal aid to detox because they nurture and calm you when you may well be feeling exhausted, possibly negative and overwrought. The remedies have a balancing effect on mind and body because they set out to counterbalance negative emotions with the positive ones they induce.

There are 39 remedies, 37 from wild flowers, one from rock water – pure water from a rocky stream – and rescue remedy, which is a combination of five plants. Rescue remedy, which you can use in moments of extreme stress, and after suffering an emotional blow or a physical accident, works just as well on animals as it does on humans.

You self-medicate by placing a drop or two using the dropper provided on your tongue, or by adding drops to spring water and then drinking it. Two especially helpful during detox are

✔ **Gorse** helps with lack of hope, the feeling that it is pointless to try or go on, and the resigned acceptance of chronic illness or difficulty. This should pep you up if at any point you feel daunted by the detox programme.

✔ **Rock water** is excellent for self-denial, a rigid outlook and purist tendencies and could help you in detox if you aim at perfection in everything that you do.

Laughing Yourself to Health

Studies into the effects of laughter, which is used for healing purposes throughout Europe and other countries, show it to have significant health benefits. A spell of laughter exercises more muscles of the body (some say all the body's muscles) than any other single occupation including lovemaking and running a marathon (this is not to say that you burn a lot of calories while laughing, just that a larger number of muscles are used). Considering that you use 56 facial muscles alone to smile, this is not difficult to believe. This is true whether you snort with mirth, roar with laughter, giggle furiously, or undergo that full-on, 'painful' laughter variety that has you bending over weeping, gives you an abdominal stitch, and at the same time is silent.

Laughter also acts directly upon the brain and the endocrine glands to release tension-breaking chemicals and counteract the negative effects of the stress hormones adrenaline and cortisol. The health benefits of laughter include:

✔ Muscular relaxation

✔ Stress reduction

✔ Aerobic exercise

✔ Mood-boosting

✔ Strengthening and balancing the immune system

✔ Enhancing confidence

✔ Natural painkiller.

If you think about it, all these are beneficial when undergoing any kind of a cleansing and balancing programme.

Try one of these methods for provoking huge laughter:

✔ Buy, borrow or replay a video or DVD that you find terribly funny, such as *Fawlty Towers*.

✔ Read the cartoon(s) in your favourite newspapers and magazines, or read your favourite humorous newspaper columnist.

✔ Buy a book of jokes and phone a friend to share the laughter. Search your brain for jokes you've been told in the past that have really made you roar with laughter. Then sit, relax and replay them on your own personal mental video.

Chapter 20

Ten Myths about Detox

*M*yths are mistaken beliefs that embed themselves in the consciousness of many people, and myths abound about detox. This is not surprising when you consider the controversy that has surrounded detox in the past when no-one really knew what it was and, more recently, with its high profile as a slimmer and beautifier of today's celebrities.

But when it comes to applying the same principles to yourself, do you not feel the odd twinge of doubt? The hype surrounding 'A-list' celebrities' health fads may make fascinating reading, but their red-carpeted, champagne-soaked, jet-transported lifestyles are hardly yours or mine.

So . . . do you believe that what works, and is apparently safe, for Liz Hurley, for example, will necessarily be so for you?

This chapter offers answers to some common myths about detox.

Detox Helps You Lose Weight Quickly

Detox diets are not primarily low calorie. What you eat and drink while detoxing will probably provide fewer calories than you usually consume if you tend to eat high-fat, high-sugar takeaways and junk snacks or convenience foods. Weight loss, however, is not the main target of the detox regimen. The main detox aim is to cleanse your liver and other eliminatory organs, and help you replace toxic habits and diet with healthier alternatives.

Detoxing does, however, set into motion various mechanisms that stimulate the breakdown of surplus fat and the loss of excess fluid. Fibre-rich, low-G.I. (glycaemic index) carbohydrates such as whole-grains, pulses, and beans release sugar into the bloodstream far more slowly than sugary snacks such as chocolate, sweets, and fizzy drinks. As a result, your insulin level falls and also becomes more sensitive to lower levels of blood sugar. Food fuel is consumed more efficiently for use by the body's tissues and organs, and inroads are made into layers of surplus fat, a percentage of which is metabolised to release energy.

During detox, salt consumption is reduced, which encourages the body to get rid of surplus fluid. More fluid is removed by the use of herbal supplements, such as dandelion, corn silk, and globe artichoke, which have a diuretic effect, increasing your urine output.

The dietary changes themselves may produce water. For every one part of fat that is eliminated, 9 parts of water are eliminated too, so some weight loss during the first few days of detox is due to fluid loss as the water is excreted. However, you will be losing fat too! More importantly, you will *feel* lighter, and your clothes looser and more comfortable.

My best advice is to focus on detox's main objective – cleansing your body of toxins – and look on any weight loss as a bonus. If you happen to be underweight, you can easily adjust your food intake to ensure that you do not lose any further pounds.

Detox Corrects the Body's pH

Your aim, some detox experts claim, is to be slightly alkaline – above 7 on the pH scale on which 7 is neutral and below 7 is acidic – the optimum state at which food is processed. Rebalancing your body's pH through a detox programme helps your body mobilise and get rid of its toxin-laden fat.

The body's required – vital – pH is 7.4, which is slightly alkaline. And the detox theorists' notion is not borne out by the facts, because the body already possesses a sophisticated and highly sensitive acid–alkaline balancing mechanism. If this is thrown out of kilter, you, your body, the whole of you, simply ceases to function. Human cellular function depends upon the pH never varying by more than the tiniest amount from the required value. In fact, metabolic acidosis and alkalosis (excess acidity and alkalinity respectively) are life-threatening conditions requiring urgent correction with appropriate medical treatment.

Detox Is a Fad Unsupported by Scientific Evidence

Is detox just a 'fad'? Certainly detox is currently newsworthy and popular, but its benefits are very real. I believe that, as a holistic self-help method, detox is here to stay. It may, indeed, like most health trends, be eclipsed by the next therapy to catch celebrities' fancy, but detox will doubtless continue to offer health-conscious people a much-needed break from the toxic lifestyle nearly inescapable in modern life.

Detox is likely, in fact, to become ever more relevant as we become increasingly under stress, as genetically modified foods sidle into our diets, and as alcohol, chocolate, junk foods, and Friday night takeaways continue to exert their appeal (to name just a few toxic sources).

It's true that there's only anecdotal evidence (so far) to support the benefits of detox. My research disclosed no scientific studies of its effects.

But detox does at least depend upon such known facts as the health hazards of dangerous chemicals in the environment and your food, and the regenerative powers of the liver and other organs. The benefits of ingesting wholesome, naturally produced foods and drinks, drinking plenty of water, getting adequate relaxation and exercise, and partaking of natural therapies and nutritional and herbal supplements are available for you to experience.

The advantages of detoxing are felt by its followers now, and may become objectively apparent in the future, when studies compare health parameters of regular detoxers with those of people following a toxic lifestyle.

Aerobic Exercise is Vital for Detox

Absolutely not! Detox is demanding enough – you are asking your body (and mind) to accept a radical change of diet and the loss of their usual pleasures such as cigarettes, alcohol, chocolate, and takeaways. Aerobic exercise would leave you exhausted, weak, and the worse for wear. Even if you are supremely fit, which most novice detoxers are not, you need to adapt to any significant diet and lifestyle change before taking your usual aerobic run or swim.

Taking gentle walks, stretching, doing undemanding yoga poses, or following t'ai chi are much more appropriate activities during detox than strenuous aerobics.

You certainly don't need 'heavy breathing' to expel toxins! Detox mobilises toxins from the liver, tissues and elsewhere, and encourages their natural expulsion. Your lungs are perfectly adapted to expel airborne impurities – aerobic exercise merely increases your depth and rate of respiration for a limited time, and there's no evidence that 20–30 minutes' vigorous activity daily (although it is recommended by many doctors for general health reasons) leaves you more toxin-free.

By all means take advantage of fresh air (as far away from toxic traffic emission fumes as possible) and take regular, deep breaths to increase the oxygen in your blood and help all the detox processes working on your behalf.

You Have to Drink Twice as Much Fluid to Help Your Kidneys Detox

No, you don't. In fact, if you are already drinking eight and ten glasses of water daily, doubling your intake could prove very harmful. Drinking too much water can cause water intoxication – the potentially fatal hyponatraemia (low blood sodium level).This is because there's too much fluid for your overworked kidneys to expel, and it enters your circulation, over-diluting your blood and tissue fluid.

You need to drink eight and ten glasses of water daily, making sure that you take them at regular intervals rather than all at once, for example at the end of the day or when exercising. Aerobic exercise is not recommended during detox, but other circumstances, which would increase your need for additional fluid, include hot weather, a fever or other illness causing excessive perspiration, and loss of excessive body fluid due to diarrhoea or vomiting.

Binge Drinking Ruins Your Liver Past the Point where Detox Can Help

Not necessarily. The liver is a resilient and very forgiving organ, and you can, in fact, abuse it for years without causing irreparable harm. There's plenty of evidence to suggest that ceasing to drink alcohol and taking a liver-supportive supplement can help to halt and even reverse alcoholic liver damage and even generate the formation of new, healthy liver cells to replace the old and damaged ones. (Chapter 3 talks about liver functions and supplements that help them.)

Assuming that you are serious about reversing liver damage, you need to act quickly. Explain your worries to your doctor and ask for blood tests – these should include liver function and a full blood count. Decide to quit alcohol for, say, six months, starting with your detox, and have the blood tests repeated at the end of this time.

It can be hard to go it alone, but you don't have to. Ask your GP about alcohol counselling, contact the AA (Alcoholics Anonymous), or pay for some private help from a cognitive behavioural therapist (CBT), a very useful technique in challenging the thoughts and emotions associated with addictive habits.

Failing with Diets Means You'll Never Stick with a Detox Programme

Look at it this way. Past failure is absolutely no guarantee of future failure. Diets in the past with which you have 'failed' may in fact have failed you. Were they unhealthy with respect to food choices or impossible to follow? Detoxing *is* demanding – but you follow the programme for a limited period only, and this book offers plenty of advice to improve both your motivation and your eating habits when detox has ended.

There is every reason to believe that your new knowledge of detox and its powers will inspire you to follow the course as laid out in this book. You have to think of your future health and body image – not of past images and failures. The current politically correct belief that there is no failure, only a learning curve, is actually true with respect to detox. Once you master the whys and wherefores of the detox process and accept that it can greatly improve your health, then you are set to start your detox programme and benefit from it to the full.

Supplements Are Not Necessary for Detox

You may not have taken dietary supplements or herbal remedies in the past, but detox is another matter. No, you do not *have* to take them to detox successfully, but supplements and herbal remedies do aid the detox process, increasing toxin elimination and strengthening the immune system. They give you a huge advantage over detoxers who do not take them.

Many different supplements are relevant to detoxing, but perhaps the kingpin is a mutlivitamin and mineral supplement full of antioxidants. You need these free radical-fighters at all times, but never more so than when releasing toxins from your body and cranking up your immune defence system to cope with more than the usual amount.

You also require a fortified immune defence system to take you on your healthier way once you've finished detox, to boost your new energy and vitality levels.

Regular Detoxing Makes it Safe to Eat, Drink, and Even Smoke as Before

Detoxing removes many toxins from your body through its cleansing action on your liver, kidneys, lungs, gut, and skin. But you waste of all your planning and effort simply to replace the toxins by returning to unhealthy habits.

Many people detox every few months, but this is usually because their first course has left them so much better and more energetic that they want to repeat and improve upon the experience!

After a detox, you're more familiar with healthier foods and with the huge scope of recipes and meals in which they can be enjoyed (see the recipes in Part V). Cutting out alcohol and smoking should also leave you aware of how much better it is possible to feel, while taking supplements regularly brings you more into tune with your body and what it feels like when firing on all cylinders!

Completing any detox programme is an achievement, and you should find that the last thing you want is to reload your body with the toxic substances you have worked so hard to eliminate.

Detox Is Only Suitable for Youngsters

Well, it depends what is meant by youngsters! If it means people in their teens and twenties, the answer is definitely 'no'! A quick look at Part IV 'Planning Your Detox', will show you how a healthy person of any age, from teens onwards, can map out a programme tailored to their personal needs.

But if by 'youngsters' we mean the young at heart, then you are partly right. It does help to feel as if you are in your twenties even when you are a good deal older, and it will make you feel more inclined to try a health and dietary plan that many still regard as a 21st century innovation.

If you are in your thirties, forties and beyond, and regard yourself as too old to alter your habits, you may not be tempted by the idea of a detox. You might fear that it's too late for healthy changes to produce any benefits. If you feel like this you may well think otherwise once you have read this book!

Chapter 21

Ten Tips to Help You Stay Motivated

In This Chapter

▶ Realising that motivation is the secret of successful detox

▶ Making sure that you can motivate yourself

▶ Knowing that you can stay motivated throughout detox

*M*otivation is the success secret behind any achievement, whether it's earning a place in the Olympic team, learning to walk again after an accident, passing your driving test, or completing a supermarket shop when you fear crowds.

Likewise, you need a motivation in order to succeed with detox, a regimen that requires changes in your diet and lifestyle. Motivation is a knack – or rather, several knacks – that you can learn, practise, and use for successful detox, as this chapter shows.

Be Specific About Your Goals

You've read about toxins within you and your surroundings, and how they can harm your health. You like the idea of being clean within and without, and knowing that your lifestyle contributes to the health of your liver, kidneys, lungs, gut, and skin.

With your personal challenges in mind, write down five changes you wish to make during detox. Opposite them, write down the benefits these changes will bring. Fix this list to a mirror or fridge where you will see it often, and make sure that you read it when you do so!

Table 21-1 offers a sample list.

Table 21-1	Sample Goals and Benefits List
Goal	**Benefits**
Quitting smoking	Breathing pure, life-giving air into increasingly healthy lungs.
Reducing alcohol consumption	A well-earned rest for your liver that allows it to channel its resources into purifying your body throughout.
Saying 'no' to junk snacks and convenience foods	The knowledge that your cholesterol and weight are on the way down, and your arteries less clogged with fatty deposits.
Reducing your sugar intake	Re-educating your taste buds to rely for sweetness on natural foods such as carrots, parsnips, sweet potatoes, fruit, and occasionally honey, which makes artificially sweetened foods easier to decline in future. Lowering your insulin levels and making your body more efficient at burning its surplus fat.
Eating more vegetables	Realising that vegetables' natural fibre, and antioxidant vitamins, minerals, and trace elements are encouraging your bowel to work regularly, clearing toxins in bile and digestive waste, leaving you with fresh breath, less bloating, and clearer skin.

Seek and Ye Shall Find . . .

. . . help. Firstly in this book, then possibly from a friend with whom to detox, an exercise partner, or a role model.

Try to find a friend – or your partner, family, a relative – to join you in your pursuit of better health. They are more likely to agree if you ask them at an appropriate time (that is, not when you're out clubbing, or one of you is rushing off to an appointment!). Assure them that,unlike a weight loss diet, a detox regimen lasts for days only, and clearly explain to them the benefits of detox.

You might also think of finding an exercise or relaxation partner (maybe your detox pal?). Gentle exercise and relaxation are important in detox and essential for improved health. Extolling the virtues of losing excess weight, eliminating loads of toxins, boosting your mood with natural highs, and dealing better with stress may well gain you an exercise companion (and morale-booster).

Your role model could be some celebrity who claims that detox has helped them achieve their flawless complexion, slim, post-birth figure, or high energy level. Alternatively, look for a role model among your friends, colleagues, or acquaintances who has benefited from detox.

Enjoy Yourself

Detox is a positive experience offering brilliant benefits, not a punishment for past misdeeds! You know which aspects of detox self-care you're going to enjoy most – delicious, healthy meals, calming relaxation, saunas and warm baths and showers, aromatherapy oils and a massage, or simply chilling out. You can intensify the pleasure by remembering that you're doing something for *yourself,* which is a positive step towards improved self-confidence. Your detox is also of help to others as your health, appearance, mood, body image, and stamina become better than ever before.

Create Goals and Rewards Along the Way

Perhaps you associate stars and bars with children's homework? Well, we're all children at heart, and the child within you needs special nurturing when you start a detox regimen. Saying no to sweets (or more adult indulgences) can cause disappointment and rebellion and the feeling that detox is just too much trouble.

First – goals. Ring the dates of your detox course on a wall calendar, in your diary and desk diary; wherever you will catch sight of them at least once a day. Then cross each day through as you complete it, sticking a gold star over it when you've taken all the detox measures you have planned, or a silver star when you strayed only once by eating a sweet or smoking one last cigarette. Your sense of achievement will grow speedily as the time passes.

Next – the rewards. If you have a strong visual imagination, seeing crossed-off detox days dotted with silver and gold stars may be reward enough. If your choice of reward is more likely to be dietary, set aside your delicious detox snacks to meet the occasion. A handful of your favourite (uncoated, unsalted) nuts, a piece of exotic fruit or some fresh bio-yoghurt scattered with seeds, are all excellent choices (sunflower seeds contain a plant constituent that helps stem nicotine cravings).

Remember That One Lost Battle Does Not Mean Defeat!

So, your positive thoughts and negative desires engaged in combat and the positive thoughts lost. A slip-up is a pity, to be avoided certainly, but it's neither the end of the world nor the end of your detox plan.

Get straight back on track by forgiving yourself (no one's perfect), making a note of the events leading up to the temptation, and jotting down a couple of ways to prevent its recurrence. This learning curve can prove most useful in future.

If stress brought you temporarily to your knees, learn the five minute relaxation technique explained in Chapter 9. If feeling deprived and in need of TLC, look at your starred calendar (see the preceding section) and remind yourself how well you are doing. Promise yourself a long, luxurious soak in an aromatherapy-scented bath (see Chapter 19 for other relaxation tips) at the next available moment.

Plan Ahead

You can keep motivated by planning your day ahead. Take packed detox lunches to work or school to avoid the temptation of junk snacks and convenience foods. If you've a long day ahead or do heavy physical work, ensure that you have sufficient complex carbohydrates (such as wholegrains, legumes, and sweet potatoes) to maintain your energy levels.

Think Pure Thoughts

Yes, of course you can think about sex! All that healthy food, fresh air and exercise, not to mention the pampering massages and aromatherapy baths are likely to put you in the mood for love. The pure thoughts I'm talking about, however, are about avoiding and getting rid of toxins.

On the food front, you can sometimes ward off an urge to eat an additive-rich piece of cake, for instance, by asking yourself: 'What would a newly detoxed person choose to do?' Think of the toxins your body is getting rid of right now, and ask yourself whether you want to slow down or even reverse these benefits.

Likewise, when remembering to drink eight to ten glasses of water every day, think of the pure water sluicing through your system, washing out toxins and accumulated debris from your gut, kidneys, and bladder.

It's harder, perhaps, to remember that stress gives rise to impurities, but the free radicals (hyperactive oxygen molecules) that develop when stress factors are high cause tissue damage and organ changes that encourage toxin damage. You may not *feel* like sipping freshly squeezed apple and/or carrot juice when your partner or family are quaffing wine or beer – just allow yourself a few superior thoughts, and picture the pure, antioxidant-rich drink mopping up the free radicals and energising your system.

Affirm Your Affirmations

Affirmations are positive statements of intent, and an invaluable tool for getting a job done.

Apt examples of affirmations include 'I can, I must, and I *will* cleanse my body of toxins,' 'Millions of people just like me have completed a detox course – I can, too,' and, especially when dealing with cravings, 'I am free of the desire for chocolates, sweets, and takeaways (or whatever). I choose a health drink/detox snack instead.'

Affirmations work on your subconscious mind so that, even though the words you are saying seem far from the truth, they actually embed themselves in your mind. Next time you're faced with a similar temptation, bingo! The repeated affirmations come into play, strengthening your sense of purpose and increasing your chances of success.

It's a good idea to come up with two or three affirmations and repeat them a dozen or so times, several times daily. Writing them down is even more effective, especially if you capitalise on this and fix the written-out sentences where you're bound to see them frequently.

Just remember to use positive statements throughout – avoid saying, for instance, 'I am not tempted to drink alcohol, or have a cigarette,' or 'I am not going to fail in my efforts to detox.' Say 'I am free from this or that temptation as in the example above,' or 'I *will* succeed in my efforts to cleanse my system.'

Track, Track, Track

Massive evidence exists that keeping a record of your progress, enhances your chances of success. Professional weight-loss companies urge their clients to keep written records of their dietary experiences from day-to-day, providing details of what they have eaten and when, how they felt before and after succumbing to temptation, and which particular stresses or negative experiences caused them to make unwise choices.

Writing things down (or recording them on a Dictaphone or video), increases your sense of purpose and provides a useful day-to-day record. Reading (listening) back over a positive and 'easy' day increases your sense of achievement and prepares you for continuing success. Reviewing a hard or challenging day when things didn't go according to plan, helps you to see minor stresses and nuisance factors in perspective and plan how best to deal with them should they recur.

Master Your Emotions

You can channel any negative feelings that arise into healthy outlets. Make sure you have food-free emotional band-aids, especially if you already have a tendency to eat whenever faced by adversity.

Use these suggestions for coping with irritation, disappointment, anger, a low mood, disappointment, boredom, and persistent anxiety and self-doubt:

- ✔ Phone a friend. Any good friend will do, and better still if he or she is either sharing detox with you or at least sympathises with what you are trying to achieve.

- ✔ Calm down and meditate. Meditate either at a pre-arranged time as described in Chapter 9, or whenever you happen to have an emergency. Chill out and still your thoughts to help deal more gracefully with unwanted pressure.

- ✔ Change your environment for an hour or so. Go for a walk in the park or fields, go swimming underwater (or just swimming), or read a book that removes you light years away from your trying surroundings.

Appendix

The Benefits of Eating Healthily

Checking Out Fruit and Veg

Everyone knows fruit and veg are good for you, but what makes them good? Here's just some of the ingredients mentioned in the recipes and the beneficial and detox-related effects each can give you.

Alfalfa sprouts: contain free radical-fighting antioxidant, especially chlorophyll. They are high in potassium, and contain some calcium.

Apples and pears: are high in vitamin C.

Asparagus: provides vitamins A and some Bs, and folate (folic acid).

Bamboo shoots: provide vitamins A, C, E, plus calcium, magnesium, and iron.

Bananas: give you sugars, fibre, and potassium.

Bean shoots: are a source of vitamins A and C.

Beetroot: cleanses the blood, is a great liver function supporter, has antiviral properties and is rich in beta-carotene and other antioxidants.

Blueberries: contain a group of antioxidants called anthrocyanides whichanthrocyanides, which are concentrated in the skin and give the fruit its blue colour. Nutritionists have identified at least 15 different anthrocyanides , and they are known to enhance micro-circulation (blood circulation in the smallest blood vessels). This helps to explain their beneficial effects upon the eyes, lungs, digestive tract, and connective tissue.

Anthrocyanides also reduce the risks of cancer, heart attacks and strokes, and age-related brain changes such as dementia, Alzheimer's disease, poor memory, poor concentration, and deficient co-ordination. Blueberries have an antibacterial action within the urinary tract, by preventing bacteria sticking to the linings of the kidneys, ureters and bladder. The recommended intake daily is around 50–75 grams – a small handful.

Blueberries (also known as bilberries in the UK and Europe) have been used for hundreds of years to protect and improve deficient eyesight, and some glaucoma sufferers have found that their sight has improved in response to eating the fruit regularly or taking a blueberry extract supplement.

Broccoli: was grown for medicinal purposes in England and other parts of Europe in medieval times, and has recently been shown to boost the immune system against cancer. Sulforaphane, one of this vegetable's most beneficial constituents, mobilises cellular enzymes (helpers) that inactivate carcinogens and other inimical substances (so should feature in all detox plans, when large quantities of toxins are expelled from the body). In fact, so much importance is attached to this broccoli phytochemical, that, in the year 2000, scientists at the John Innes Centre in Norwich, UK, created a non-genetically modified super-broccoli containing up to 100 times more sulforaphane by crossing the common or garden version with its wild Sicilian cousin. Broccoli also contains isothiocynates, which trigger the manufacture of the body's own cancer-fighting substances, and inhibit cellular growth in the skin cancer, melanoma. Another constituent, indole-3-carbinol, cuts the risks of hormone-related cancers of the breast, prostate, and ovaries.

Capers: contain calcium, magnesium, and vitamins A, E, and some Bs.

Carrots: are a very popular vegetable and are good for beta-carotene and other antioxidant carotenoids that fight cancer. They are also good as a source of potassium, calcium, protein, and carbohydrates, mainly natural sugars.

Celery: has sodium and potassium content, which make it an excellent diuretic, and compounds known as phthalides in celery reduce both blood pressure (you need to eat four stalks a day!), and cholesterol. Celery's coumarin compounds have antioxidant effects, helping to combat cancer. It is also an excellent source of vitamin C (one of the most potent antioxidants), and also of vitamin B2 (riboflavin), vitamin A (beta-carotene), fibre, manganese and iron. Additionally, celery supplies the amino acid tryptophan (which is needed for serotonin production in the brain – a mood chemical), vitamin B6 (pyridoxine), potassium, manganese, and molybdenum. Other benefits include magnesium, calcium, vitamin B1, and folate (the natural form of folic acid, needed for healthy blood cell production and the health of unborn babies.)

Chinese gooseberries: (Kiwi fruit) contain vitamin C, and a little calcium, iron, and vitamin A.

Chives: are a source of calcium and iron, plus all the major vitamins: A, Bs, C, E, and K.

Cucumbers: provide potassium, magnesium, vitamin C, and folate.

Figs: give you potassium, calcium, iron, vitamin C, fructose, glucose, soluble and insoluble fibre.

Garlic: may not be everyone's favourite, especially after it's eaten by others, but it does contains antioxidants, as well as thinning blood, and reducing harmful cholesterol.

Grapefruit flesh/juice: provides vitamin C, bioflavonoids (from the scraped pith and membranes), fibre, a little protein and complex carbohydrates, and it is virtually fat-free. Grapefruit is also an excellent source of potassium.

Green beans: are good for providing vitamin C, potassium, and manganese.

Green pepper: contains antioxidant chlorophyll; it supplies trypto-phan amino acid, and vitamin B6; and vitamins beta-carotene (A), K, thiamine B1 (prescribed during medical detox – see Chapter 4); folate (folic acid), which aids blood cell formation and healthy growth of unborn babies; fibre; trace element molybdenum, low levels of which have been linked to depression in a number of people.

Lemon juice: contains citric acid, a natural bacteria-killer (bacte-ricidal). It also contains antioxidants, including vitamin C, and bioflavonoids.

Lemon peel: although not strictly that edible by itself, it does contain some vitamin C and is rich in bioflavonoids, powerful antioxidants that enhance vitamin C's actions in the body. They are an ideal nutritional source during the detox process.

Lychees: are a source of fibre, vitamin C, and potassium.

Melon: gives you potassium, zinc, selenium, iron, range of B vitamins, vitamin E, folic acid, beta-carotene, and vitamin C.

Onions: provide complex carbs, fibre, potassium, and calcium.

Oranges: contain just under 200 active plant constituents, the best known of which are vitamin C and bioflavonoids. These two powerful anxtioxidants work together to protect various organs and tissues against cancer, inflammation, infection, blood clots, and fatty deposits that clog arteries. They also reduce the risks of flu, colds, and other infections as well as asthma, arthritis, strokes, thrombosis, high blood pressure, and arterial disease. Other disorders thought to benefit from eating oranges include macular degeneration (an age-related eye disease that can cause blindness), dementia, gallstones, diabetes, cataracts, and gingivitis (gum inflammation).

Parsnips: give you potassium, fibre, complex carbs, vitamins B3, C, and E.

Paw paw (papaya): contains protein, fibre, complex carbohydrates, vitamin C and folic acid. Papaya also contains papain digestive enzymes.

Pomegranate seeds: known as 'the jewels of winter', possibly because of their connection with Pluto, King of the Hades underworld (synonymous with winter), and Persephone, Goddess of Spring. They are three times as rich in antioxidants as red wine and green tea and also provide potassium, vitamin C, fibre and niacin (vitamin B3), needed by the nervous system.

Raspberries: provide vitamin C, ellargic acid, calcium, iron, fibre, protein, and fruit sugars.

Redcurrants or white currants: good for fibre, fruit sugars, vitamins A and C, iron, calcium, and potassium.

Spinach: is famous for containing iron as all of you who know about Popeye will remember. It also contains other minerals including potassium, magnesium, manganese, vitamin C, and bioflavonoids, and folate.

Spring greens/cabbage: are great as a source of soluble fibre, calcium, potassium, vitamins A, C and B group, and folic acid. They contain antioxidants, and their isothiocyanates and sulfurophane have cancer-fighting properties. Cabbage's 'vitamin U' (not actually a true vitamin) combats stomach inflammation and peptic ulcer pain.

Strawberries: as well as providing vitamin C, also contains two powerful cancer-fighting flavonoids, quercetin and kaempferol, and another cancer-fighting phytonutrient, ellargic acid.

Tomatoes: and tomato puree are good for vitamin C, beta-carotene (provitamin A), lycopene – an antioxidant, bright-red phytochemical found in tomatoes (and guavas, watermelon and pink grapefruit) with powerful cancer-beating properties, especially of the prostate gland. Concentration in puree, ketchups etc, and heating during cooking, increase lycopene's availability to the body.

It's Not Just Fruit and Veg

Also valuable when detoxing are mushrooms, nuts, spices, and the many herbs that are readily available. And don't forget seaweed and soy sauce from Japanese cuisine. They all add flavour and texture to detox recipes to make them even more appealing while staying healthy.

Basil: may relieve headaches and hangovers. It also contains vitamin C and chlorophyll.

Bay leaf: contains the antioxidant chlorophyll; essential oils from this herb aid the release of stomach wind, improve poor digestion and help to clear the chest of phlegm.

Bio yoghurt: contains healthy bacteria, calcium.

Black pepper: promotes the body's fat-burning ability.

Bonito flakes: are rich in protein, especially the amino acids methionine, lysine, and tyrosine, which are involved in the production of the natural mood-lifting nerve messenger, serotonin, in the brain. Rich in omega-3 essential fatty acids, bonito also provides the fat-soluble vitamins A, D, E and K, many of the B complex vitamins, and minerals calcium, sodium, and iron.

Caraway seeds: are low in sodium and fats and supply calcium, vitamins A and C, and iron.

Chicory: provides potassium, calcium, and vitamin C.

Cider vinegar: is rich in minerals such as potassium and antioxidants. It also contains calcium, and vitamins A, Bs, C, and E.

Cinnamon: settles the stomach.

Cumin seeds: are very rich in iron, needed for the haemoglobin molecule in red blood cells which transports oxygen throughout the body. Pregnant and breast-feeding women, as well as growing children and adolescents, are especially in need of iron supplies.

Cumin seeds are also powerful antioxidants, with cancer-defeating actions. They stimulate the release of pancreatic enzymes, essential to a healthy digestion, and are mentioned in the Bible as valuable currency for paying tithes to priests. They were greatly valued in ancient Rome and Greece, because applying the ground seeds to the face causes the complexion temporarily to pale – an effect exploited by students to convince their tutors that they had been burning the midnight oil.

Coconut: is good for fibre, potassium, calcium, and complex carbohydrates.

Fennel: adds a delicious flavour to recipes in which it is included. It is rich in fibre, calcium, potassium, folate and both manganese and molybdenum. It also provides calcium, manganese, iron, phosphorus, magnesium, and vitamin B3.

Ginger: has a reputation for soothing gastrointestinal disorders. Ginger has been shown to offer protection against colo-rectal cancer, and to provide supplies of potassium, magnesium, copper, manganese and vitamin B6 (pyridoxine). It also has anti-inflammatory effects, and it helps to soothe gastrointestinal disorders, including peptic ulcers, heartburn, hiatus hernia, and proven peptic ulceration.

Goat's cheese: provides calcium, protein, vitamins B3 and B6, and essential fatty acids.

Honey: is bactericidal and slows down absorption of natural sugar, minimising 'sugar rush'.

Japanese soy sauce: (shoyu) is made from cooked soya beans, roasted and crushed wheat, and brine. Even so, shoyu contains less salt (sodium) than the Chinese variety. For main benefits, see Tofu. Also look for *salt-reduced shoyu,* and for *tamari,* made with such tiny quantities of wheat that it is recommended as gluten-free for people with coeliac disease and other forms of wheat intolerance.

Lentils: are especially rich in molybdenum. They also supply folate, fibre, essential proteins, the amino acid tryptophan, vitamin B1 (thiamine), as well as iron, copper, manganese, phosphorus, and vitamin B1 (thiamine) – essential to the brain and nervous system.

Mint: provides a wide range of oxidants, and recent research has indicated that it can kill cancerous cells.

Molasses: comprises sugars, and sulphur, and is very rich in potassium and calcium.

Mushrooms: contain vitamin B5 (pantothenate), boost energy and wound healing, and combat fatigue and the adverse and toxic effects of most antibiotics. Field mushrooms also provide zinc, selenium, and vitamin B2 (riboflavin), which help to promote growth and reproduction, and healthy nails, hair, and skin. Vitamin B2 also benefits vision, alleviating eye fatigue, and acts with other essential nutrients to metabolise carbohydrates, fats and proteins. There are reports that mushrooms also help to reduce the risks of breast cancer.

Mustard powder: has zinc, protein, calcium, and potassium.

Nutmeg: aids the digestion and relieves queasiness.

Oats: are great nerve soothers. Oats and oat bran significantly reduce blood levels of cholesterol, and aid sugar balance in diabetics.

Olive oil: contains cholesterol-lowering mono-unsaturated fatty acids, potassium, and calcium.

Parsley: acts as a diuretic, increasing toxin loss in the urine. It is rich in calcium and iron and its chlorophyll content combats detox bad breath, and boosts the oxygen-transporting capabilities of the blood; this purifies the blood, increasing the oxygen supply to all the major organs.

Poppy seeds: give you fibre, polyunsaturates, calcium, and potassium.

Sultanas/raisins/currants: provide sugars, fibre, vitamins, and minerals.

Tofu is curd made from soya bean milk. It's an excellent source of protein, including tryptophan, and rich in omega-3 fatty acids, calcium, magnesium, phosphorus and copper, iron, manganese, and selenium. Recent research has shown that regular intakes of soya, including tofu, can lower total cholesterol by up to 30 per cent and the dangerous type (LDL) by between 35 and 40 per cent. It also reduces triglyceride levels and the blood's tendency to form dangerous clots (thrombosis.) Tofu also contains phyto-oestrogens, especially the isoflavones genistein and diadzein, which act as very, very weak oestrogens, relieving menopausal symptoms such as hot flushes and sweats, and the tendency to develop osteoporosis. (Many forms of tofu are also calcium-enriched, increasing the protection against this bone-thinning disease.)

Turmeric: contains anti-inflammatory antioxidant, which boosts liver function and bile secretion (aiding detox), helps damaged liver cells to regenerate, and combats blood clotting and raised cholesterol levels.

Watercress: provides minerals including iron, beta-carotene (provitamin A), vitamin C and bioflavonoids plus other antioxidants including chlorophyll. It also provides magnesium, zinc, and iron.

Wakame: and most edible seaweeds, are fat and cholesterol-free, and provide small quantities of carbohydrates and protein, including the amino acid tryptophan. Their main essential nutrients include calcium, magnesium, manganese, iron and zinc, and vitamins A, C, B complex riboflavin, niacin and pantothenic acid, folate, and vitamin K. Kelp is rich in iodine, and may help body fat loss caused by an underactive thyroid.

Walnuts: give you omega-3 oils and fibre.

Index

• **S** •

Notes

Notes

Notes

Notes

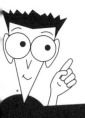

FOR DUMMIES®

Do Anything. Just Add Dummies

UK editions

...ME

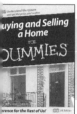

...uying and Selling a Home

0-7645-7027-7

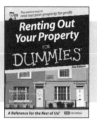

Renting Out Your Property

0-470-02921-8

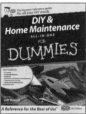

DIY & Home Maintenance ALL-IN-ONE

0-7645-7054-4

...SONAL FINANCE

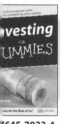

...vesting

7645-7023-4

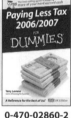

Paying Less Tax 2006/2007

0-470-02860-2

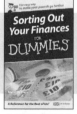

Sorting Out Your Finances

0-7645-7039-0

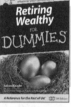

Retiring Wealthy

0-470-02632-4

...INESS

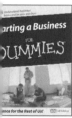

...arting a Business

-7645-7018-8

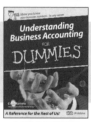

Understanding Business Accounting

0-7645-7025-0

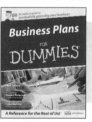

Business Plans

0-7645-7026-9

...LTH & PERSONAL DEVELOPMENT

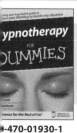

...ypnotherapy

-470-01930-1

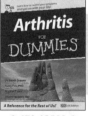

Nutrition

0-7645-7058-7

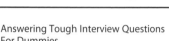

Arthritis

0-470-02582-4

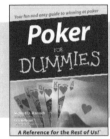
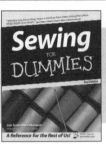
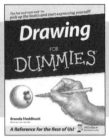
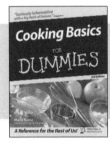
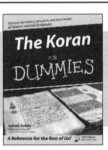
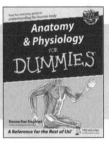
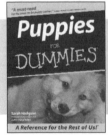
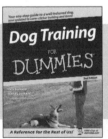
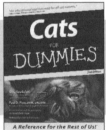

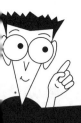

FOR DUMMIES

Do Anything. Just Add Dummies

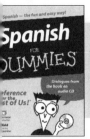
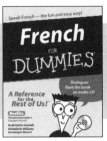
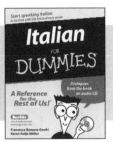
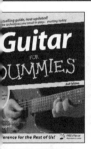
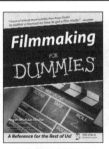
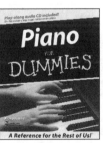
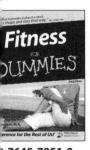
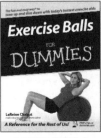
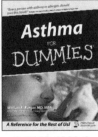

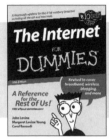
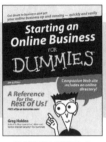
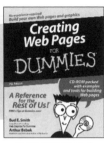
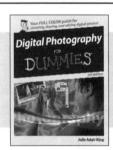
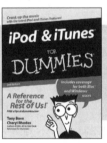
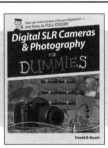
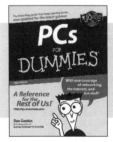
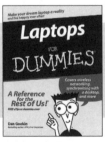
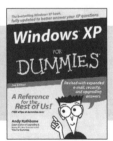